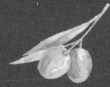

THE OLIVE OIL
& SEA SALT
COMPANION

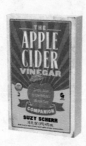
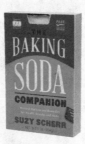
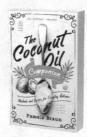
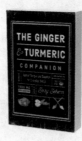
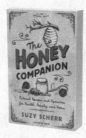

THE OLIVE OIL & SEA SALT COMPANION

100 RECIPES AND REMEDIES FROM THE PANTRY

SUZY SCHERR

THE COUNTRYMAN PRESS

A Division of W. W. Norton & Company

Independent Publishers Since 1923

This book is intended as a general information resource. It is not a substitute for professional advice and no recommendation in this book to eat, drink, or use anything is intended to substitute for any prescribed medication. While sea salt has some beneficial properties that table salt does not, both pose the same health risks, and there are individuals sensitive to both. Sea salt does not contain iodine, which is an essential nutrient. Consult your healthcare provider before changing your diet in any significant way and in particular before ingesting significant amounts of salt or olive oil, especially if you have high blood pressure or kidney disease, are taking prescribed medications, are diabetic or suffer from any other health condition, are pregnant or nursing, or have food or other allergies, such as allergies to olives. Do the same before you offer any new foods, ingredients, or products to children or use aerosol products around children. If any of the products in this book do not alleviate the condition for which you ate or took it, consult your doctor.

For information about permission to reproduce selections
from this book, write to Permissions, The Countryman Press,
500 Fifth Avenue, New York, NY 10110

For information about special discounts for bulk purchases,
please contact W. W. Norton Special Sales at
specialsales@wwnorton.com or 800-233-4830

Manufacturing by Versa Press
Production Manager: Gwen Cullen

Library of Congress Cataloging-in-Publication Data

Names: Scherr, Suzy, author.
Title: The olive oil & sea salt companion : 100 recipes and remedies from
  the pantry / Suzy Scherr.
Other titles: The olive oil and sea salt companion
Description: New York, NY : The Countryman Press, [2021] | Series:
  Countryman pantry series | Includes index.
Identifiers: LCCN 2021013870 | ISBN 9781682686300 (pbk) | ISBN
  9781682686317 (epub)
Subjects: LCSH: Cooking (Olive oil) | Sea salt. | LCGFT: Cookbooks.
Classification: LCC TX819.O42 S4 2021 | DDC 641.6/463—dc23
LC record available at https://lccn.loc.gov/2021013870

The Countryman Press
www.countrymanpress.com

A division of W. W. Norton & Company, Inc.
500 Fifth Avenue, New York, NY 10110
www.wwnorton.com

10 9 8 7 6 5 4 3 2 1

In memory of my dad

CONTENTS

MAINS

HEALING TREATMENTS

BEAUTY SECRETS

HOUSEHOLD USES

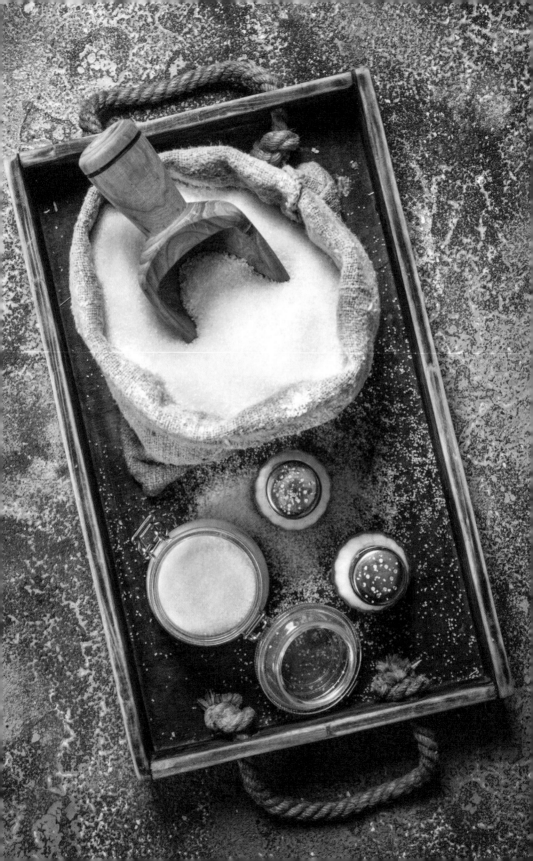

INTRODUCTION

Olive oil and sea salt. They're two of the most common kitchen staples around. You've probably used olive oil in a dressing here or there or dipped a crusty hunk of baguette into a golden puddle of the stuff. Or maybe you're like me, a devotee to the core, treating it as your go-to for all manner of cooking from sautés to pastas to roasted dishes and even baked goods. But maybe not. Maybe you're like a lot of cooks for whom olive oil isn't the oil of choice. (Well, not yet, anyway.) And what about sea salt? For many of us, using salt means wielding a shaker over a pot or a plate a couple of times and considering a food seasoned "to taste." End of story. But it *isn't* the end of the story—believe me, there's much more to tell.

So, where does it begin? I'm a chef, so if you ask me (and by picking up this book, I suppose you just did), the story *always* starts in the kitchen. There, olive oil (specifically extra virgin— more on that distinction later) and sea salt are pretty much the building blocks of all good food. They're kitchen "basics," yes, but they are also ingredients that—if used in just the right way—will make your food stand out, pop, and sparkle. Together or separately, olive oil and sea salt are indispensable and powerful, and I absolutely cannot imagine cooking without either one of them. To put it another way, olive oil and sea salt are a bit like Diana Ross and Lionel Richie. They're both amazing, celebrated, iconic artists. But unite them, and what do you get? You get "Endless Love," the greatest duet of all time and the biggest number one hit for either artist! Olive oil and sea salt each bring something different, something big to the table—but use them together and they make magic happen.

Culinary magic aside, I don't wear my chef hat all day—I'm a busy mom and wife, with a never-ending to-do list and not enough hours in the day. I need all the help I can get to steer this ship to shore and, at the risk of mixing metaphors, olive oil and sea salt are my life preservers. They do wonders well beyond the four imperfect, glitter glue– and construction paper–decorated walls of my kitchen. They are the ingredients I rely on daily to improve and maintain my family's health, to clean our house, and to make my skin glow. (Hang on. Nope, that "glow" is actually sweat from my 75th trip down the stairs to simultaneously help with math homework and locate a missing stuffed animal. Trust me, though, olive oil and sea salt are amazing for your skin.)

And when I say that they do "wonders" outside the kitchen, what I mean is that they are multitasking superstars. Sea salt—all at once antiseptic, softening, smoothing, and oil-absorbing—is great for the skin, for dental hygiene, and in self-care products that contribute to overall wellness. It's indispensable around the house—one of those endlessly versatile ingredients that works as a go-to part of any green cleaning arsenal. And ingesting appropriate amounts of salt provides you with trace minerals; prevents dehydration; promotes brain, nervous system and muscle function; supports digestive health; and promotes nutrient absorption. Plus, it can help with conditions ranging from fatigue and adrenal disorders to blood pressure and cholesterol levels.

Olive oil, meanwhile, has been credited with everything from reducing type 2 diabetes and preventing strokes to fighting depression, osteoporosis, and certain kinds of cancer. It has anti-inflammatory properties as well as fatty acids that can help to protect the brain from the toxic substances that may lead to Alzheimer's disease. Plus it's one of the most hydrating products you can put on your skin or hair, and it has been proven to prevent signs of premature aging and sun damage (after you have been out in the sun, that is). Go ahead, see whether you can find one other thing in your kitchen that can simultaneously quiet a squeaky door; give you gorgeous, shiny hair; soothe a sore throat; lower your risk of heart disease; and help you get dinner made. No chance.

This book will walk you through many of the easy and accessible ways in which I use olive oil and sea salt every single day to nurture and care for myself and my family. My hope is that it will inspire you to cook great food and give you some simple tools for staying healthy, saving time, and finding joy and ease in your everyday life.

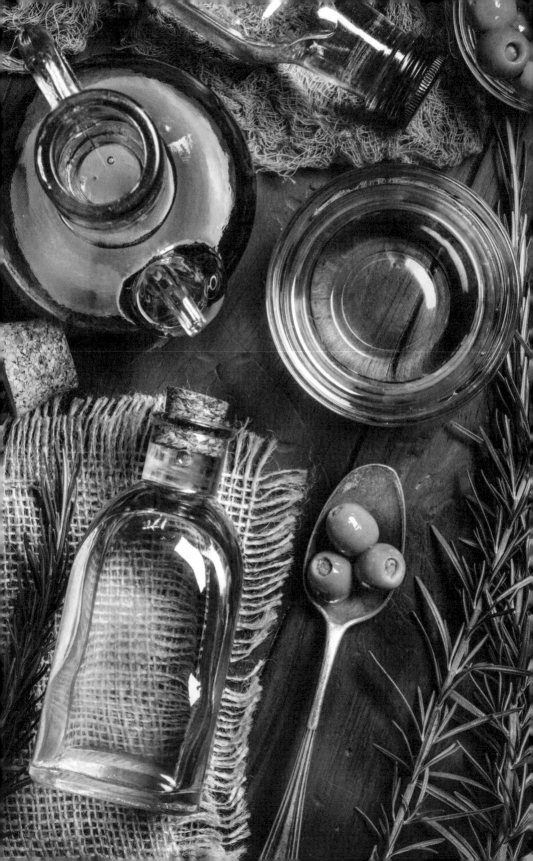

PART I

GETTING STARTED WITH OLIVE OIL AND SEA SALT

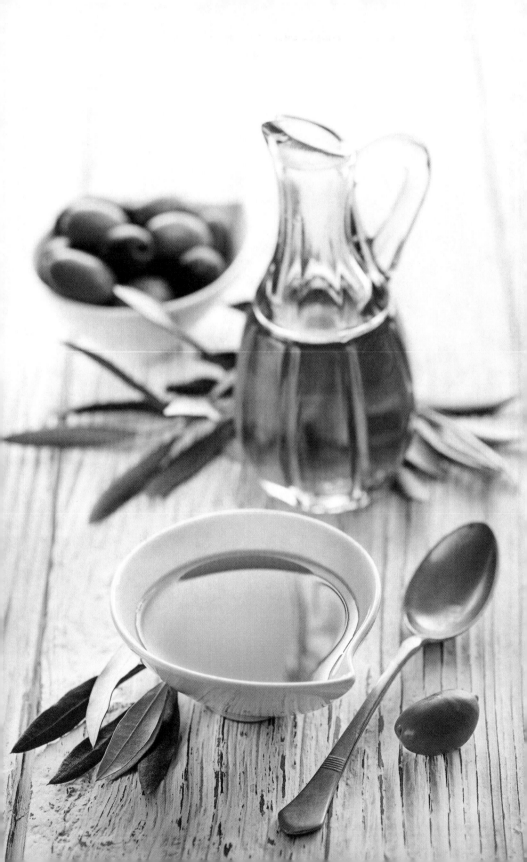

MEET OLIVE OIL

Olive Oil 101

Olive oil is my go-to fat. Yes, I have a go-to fat. And I'm sure you do, too, if you stop and think about it. It brings so much more to the table than any other fat or oil I can think of. Of course, there's a time and a place for canola and vegetable oils. And butter? I *get* butter, believe me! But olive oil is something else. It tastes great, can be used on pretty much *anything*—not just food, of course, because, as we know, there are loads of beauty and household uses for olive oil, too—and it has health benefits out the wazoo.

But What Is It?

In the most basic terms, olive oil is fruit juice. When olives—the fruit of the olive tree—are crushed, olive oil is extracted. That's it, really. That's olive oil.

Of course, there are all kinds of olive oils that come from many different types of olives. And there are various grades of olive oils, too. We'll get into the varieties and the reason that I refer mainly to extra virgin olive oil for the purposes of this book, but for now, know that what distinguishes olive oil from most other oils is the fact that it is extracted from the whole fruit, rather than from a seed or nut.

A Very Long History, Very Briefly

Suffice it to say olive oil has been around for a very, very long time. Olive trees have grown wild in the Mediterranean for tens of thousands of years and were the first plants to be actively cultivated there. It's no wonder, then, that much of the world's olive oil still comes from such countries as Greece, Spain, and Italy. That's where its history runs deepest. Since Homer was the first to call it "liquid gold" and winners of the Olympic Games in ancient Greece brought it home as their victory prize, olive oil has long been considered one of life's treasures—not just for its culinary virtues but also as medicine, a beauty aid, and an important part of religious rituals.

One of the Western world's most mythical, powerful, and alluring ingredients, olive oil has been shaping civilization for the last 10,000 years. The depth and importance of olive oil's antiquity and the hugeness of the mark it has made on civilization is beyond significant. So, it's rather amazing that American kitchens didn't really come to meet olive oil until roughly the 1980s, where it would be used only occasionally—and sparingly. Fast-forward another 35 years or so and, today, the market for olive oil is massive, by comparison. It's produced all over the world—from Greece, Spain, and Italy to California, Georgia, and Texas—and is used more and more as an all-purpose cooking oil.

Health Benefits

Part of the reason for olive oil's rise in popularity is our increased knowledge of its health benefits. Extra virgin olive oil, in particular, is recognized as one of the world's healthiest oils—thanks to a laundry list of healthy fats, antioxidants, and polyphenols—and research suggests that people who live in regions where olive oil is a diet staple live longer.

Science tells us that a 15-milliliter (1-tablespoon) serving of extra virgin olive oil contains approximately 135 calories and roughly 14 grams of fat. About 75 percent of that fat is oleic acid, an antioxidant and monounsaturated fat, which is associated with multiple health benefits, cardiovascular

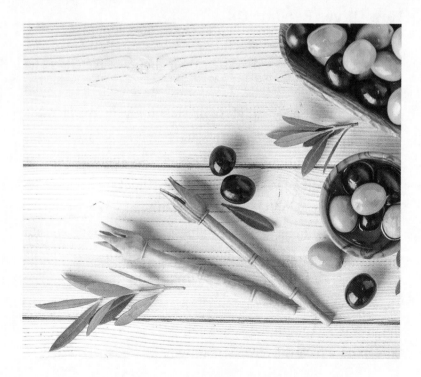

health being the most heavily documented among them. But mounting research suggests that olive oil may also improve insulin sensitivity, which helps protect against and manage type 2 diabetes. And emerging evidence linking the consumption of olive oil to a reduced risk of bone loss in old age, protection against some cancers, and the obstruction of compounds responsible for Alzheimer's disease and dementia is among some of the most promising new research out there. What's more, some studies have even found that one of the specific antioxidant compounds found in olive oil, oleocanthal, shares the same pharmacological activity as ibuprofen, making it a powerful natural anti-inflammatory.

How Olives Become Oil

You'll notice that throughout this book I almost always refer to "extra virgin olive oil," rather than simply "olive oil." (The exception is when using it around the house for things such as oiling an old baseball glove or cleaning your refrigerator doors, in which case antioxidants and polyphenols aren't going to make a bit of difference.) The reason has to do with the fact that extra virgin olive oil is produced without the application of heat, which would destroy its nutritional integrity. So, to get the biggest bang for your wellness buck, when it comes to using olive oil, extra virgin olive oil is the way to go.

Knowing how olive oil is produced is the best way to understand why this is the case. For the most part, all olive oil production starts out in the autumn or winter, depending on the climate in which the olives are grown, which is when they're harvested and then quickly milled. In the old days, olives were pressed to extract their oil, but today the process of getting olives and their oil from the branch to the bottle can happen in one of two ways and, depending on which method is used, has a direct impact on the quality and grade of the resulting oil.

- Unrefined olive oils are produced without any chemical or heat extraction processes. Instead, they are simply crushed in large metal machines, where they are turned into a paste and later transferred to a centrifuge that separates the oil from everything else. If it's any consolation, it's not the quaint image I had in my mind either, of a little old Italian grandma collecting olives in her apron and lovingly squeezing them in her own hillside olive press, but it is a simple process that results in a very high-quality product.
- Refined olive oils, on the other hand, undergo a second production after the first crushing. This next step often includes the use of heat and/or chemicals and solvents. The resulting oil is colorless and tasteless and lacks a distinct character; this inferior oil is sometimes blended with virgin olive oil (for better color and flavor).

You might think, So, there are just two types of olive oil, then? That's easy!

Well . . . not quite.

Selecting and buying olive oil can be complicated and downright overwhelming. From the country of origin and types of olives used to the processing method and the grade of the oil, there's a lot to consider when selecting olive oil. One place to start is by considering olive oil's grades.

Extra virgin olive oil is considered the top grade of olive oil, delivering the truest olive taste and most complete health benefits. This is the good stuff and this is what I suggest you use almost all of the time. To produce it, olives are crushed and the oil is extracted by mechanical means only, rather than refined through the use of heat or chemicals. Specific labeling requirements vary from country to country, but all extra virgin oil must pass a battery of chemical requirements (its oleic acid level may not surpass 0.8%) set by the International Olive Council (IOC). In addition, extra virgin olive oil undergoes rigorous smell and taste tests to ensure that there are no defects in the product. The end result is a flavorful oil with a distinct olive flavor, often a bit of spiciness, and a color that sits somewhere between golden yellow and dark green.

Virgin olive oil is a pure oil made using the same mechanical process as extra virgin olive oil, but production standards are not quite as rigid. In addition, virgin olive oil is permitted to have a slightly higher oleic acid level and typically imparts a slightly less intense flavor than extra virgin olive oil. That said, virgin olive oil has good flavor and minimal flaws.

Pure olive oil/olive oil is—for lack of a better term—"regular" olive oil. It is typically a blend of virgin olive oil and olive oil that's been chemically refined to remove any defects that have come to light in the testing process. As such, it is a lower-quality oil, with less flavor, and an oleic acid level somewhere in the neighborhood of 3 to 4 percent.

Light olive oil is really a marketing term more than anything. It's a highly refined oil that is produced using heat and/or chemicals. It often has other types of vegetable oils added to the mix as well, resulting in an overall lower-quality oil.

How to Taste It

I want you to buy high-quality olive oil because it's good for you, but more than anything, I want you to like the way it tastes. So, how do you select an oil that's going to make you happy? The best way, of course, is to taste it before you buy it. Many specialty stores will allow you to do just that, which will, of course, help you discover which styles you like best. But you can't very well help yourself to a sip here and a slurp there when cruising the olive oil aisle at the grocery store, so keep the following in mind when selecting olive oil:

As with wine, the way olive oil tastes is impacted by a number of factors, including varietal, climate, soil, and weather. Literally dozens of olive varieties are used to make olive oil around the world, and the resulting flavors and aromas can be all over the map (*get it?*)—from fruity or peppery, to bitter, herbaceous, buttery, or grassy. Knowing which olives were used to make a given oil will help you determine what the oil might taste like. In almost ridiculously simplistic terms, Italian olives tend to be more peppery and bitter, Spanish olives are often more balanced, and Greek olives are inclined to be on the fruitier side. Of course, there's much more to it than that; I encourage you to do your research, explore the many varieties of olives out there—from Koroneiki to Arbequina and everything in between—and ultimately, go with what tastes good to you. Once you've figured that out, use that oil with abandon. Use it every day for *all* of your cooking, baking and, yes, even for deep-frying. (It has a smoke point of about 400°F, so no reason not to!)

How to Buy and Store It

If you take nothing else away from this section, remember this: olive oil is a perishable product—heat, light, and air are its enemies. And, unlike wine, olive oil doesn't get better with age, so you want to buy oil as close to its bottling date as possible. If you can, buy from a producer that prints a harvest date on its label; that way, you know exactly how old the oil is when you purchase it. Unfortunately, many large producers do not label their bottles with a harvest date, but most small producers do—all the more reason to support them! And while all European producers are required by law to provide a "best by" date on the label, they don't have to disclose how old the oil was when it was bottled, so it's not terribly useful information. The USDA doesn't require date labeling of any kind, so again—finding a producer that voluntarily labels its bottles with either a bottling date or harvest date is a really good way to ensure the freshness of your oil.

To make your olive oil last, store it in a cool, dark place. Ideally, it's been sold to you in a dark bottle, which will have offered protection from light even before it arrived in your hands. If not, no worries—you can easily wrap the bottle in foil to protect it in your home. If handled properly, you can expect extra virgin olive oil to last for about 18 months.

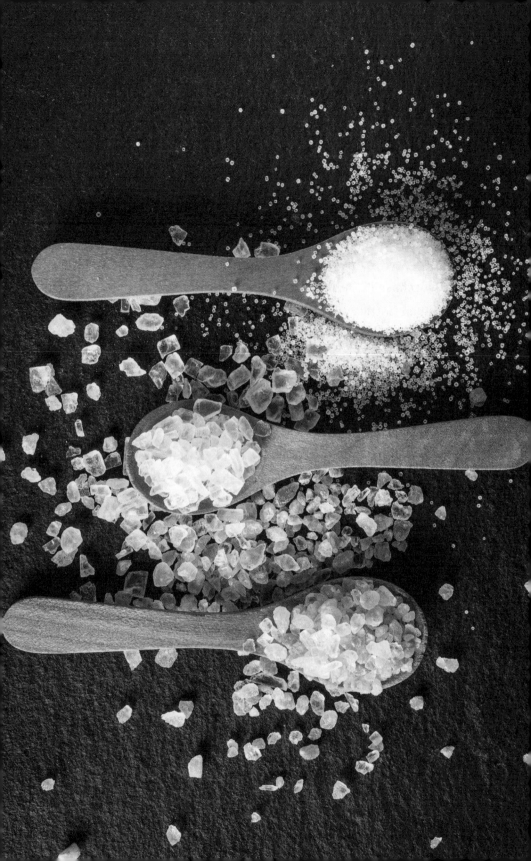

MEET SEA SALT

Sea Salt 101

Salt is the only ingredient I know of that can enhance food to make it taste ... well, *more*. More like itself—richer, meatier, even sweeter. Salt is the ingredient that melds together elements of a dish into a finished product that is the perfect balance of flavor and intensity. A touch of salt will reduce a dish's bitterness but pump up its sweet, sour, and umami qualities. A bit more salt will tamp down a food's sweetness and enhance its umami. It doesn't add flavor of its own so much as bring out the best flavor in other foods. In other words, salt is pretty much the backbone of everything delicious.

But it's not *just about* flavor when it comes to salt. Salt crystals contain trace elements needed for our very survival, which is likely why humans crave salty foods. Sea salt, in particular, which is evaporated from—you guessed it—the sea, retains more of its natural minerals than other types of salts, making it especially good for us and, therefore, useful in all sorts of home remedies. Adding it as a regular part of your diet provides a great way to enjoy good food and good health.

But What Is It?

Chemically speaking, salt is a very simple compound made up of sodium (Na) and chlorine (Cl). NaCl. Ring a bell? That high school chemistry is coming back to you now! And while it's all just sodium chloride on paper, table salt is not the same as kosher salt, which is not the same as sea salt. Sea salt is a type of salt produced from the evaporation of seawater—either by open-air solar evaporation or by a quicker process called vacuum evaporation. The result is a salt that retains traces of health-promoting minerals as well as natural flavors and colors that make it not only delicious, but a mainstay for health and wellness. (Note, however, that sea salt does not contain iodine, which is an essential health nutrient.)

A Very, Very Long History (Very Briefly)

Explaining the history of salt is a bit like trying to explain the history of everything. After all, what's older than the sea itself? Nothing. And because human bodies need sodium to survive, our history with salt goes as far back as our mere existence.

Salt's history is dizzyingly broad. From commerce and religion to medicine and, of course, cooking, we have depended on and revered salt for millennia. But salt was not always as plentiful and readily available as it is today, so it was incredibly valuable in ancient civilizations. So valuable, in fact, that at times it was taxed, minted into coins, traded on the black market, and fought over in wars. Even the word *salary* derives from the Latin word for salt.

IF YOU'RE WONDERING ABOUT TABLE SALT . . .

Table salt is a highly processed food product. Mined from salt deposits in the earth, it is always refined to remove any leftover minerals and contaminants, and is usually combined with iodine and/or anticaking agents. It's therefore not surprising, that the vast majority of salt that's added to fast food, junk food, and processed food is this highly processed table salt and not sea salt.

The earliest man first discovered the culinary importance of naturally formed salt crystals and, somehow, amazingly, figured out how to use it with food—first for curing and preserving fish and meats, and later, in the baking of bread. In all likelihood, salt-preserved foods are what allowed for the emergence of the very first trade networks, bringing with them cultural exploration, culinary complexity, and discovery. In short, salt was what helped people evolve from living a primitive life to one in which they could think strategically about their survival and the greater world around them.

Over time, our relationship with salt has become sophisticated and complex—both for better and for worse. On the one hand, industrialized food production has had an incredible and unfortunate impact on how much salt we consume. Packaged, processed food products are full of sodium (not to mention fat and sugar)—much more than we need to keep our body functioning well—and have been prime contributors to many negative health conditions around the world. On the other hand, sea salt has brought great benefit to the modern world, making its way into our diets through a booming industry of artisan salts, offering an amazing variety of top-notch, health-promoting products available to consumers all over the world.

Health Benefits

Salt is an interesting subject within the context of health. I don't know about you, but after many years of hearing that too much salt was a no-no, I had a hard time wrapping my brain around the idea that some salt could be not only good for me, but something I actually couldn't live without. Sodium can help with muscle activity, nerve stimulation, and adrenal function. Chloride supports the digestive system and proper brain functioning and growth. Plus salt contains magnesium, which is critical for nerve transmission and bone formation and may help your body resist heart disease.

But doesn't too much salt cause high blood pressure and other health problems? Well, yes and no. Excess amounts of salt *can* cause hypertension, the precursor to heart disease and stroke. This is more likely to happen in people who are genetically predisposed to have a sensitivity to salt. (You should consult your doctor to make sure you are not one of those people and also just generally to find out how much salt is right for you.)

The fact is we all need *some* salt in our diet. As long as you get your iodine from other sources, choosing unrefined sea salt—a natural product that hasn't been stripped of its beneficial trace minerals (such as calcium, potassium, magnesium, zinc, and iron) and other naturally occurring nutrients is a great way to meet that need.

The minerals in sea salt, which are electrolytes, help regulate your body's fluid balance, which in turn keeps you from becoming dehydrated. Those minerals also help promote the proper transmission of electrical signals in the body, which impacts your heartbeat, muscle function, and the overall health of your brain and nervous system. Not only that—sea salt may help your digestive system function properly. Insufficient sodium can lead to a reduction of hydrochloric acid (HCl) in your stomach, and that could, in turn, lead to an unfortunate potpourri of stomach issues, such as heartburn, stomach pain, vomiting, and constipation. And, of course, having a properly functioning digestive system with healthy levels of stomach acid is critical to the proper absorption of important vitamins and minerals, including calcium, zinc, iron, folate, and vitamin B_{12}.

Demystifying Sea Salt

At first glance, sea salt seems like the simplest ingredient around. I mean, it's *just* salt. How complicated could it be? Well, when you consider the fact that not all sea salt is harvested in the same way and not all harvesting produces the same kind of salt, things start to get a little thorny. And when you delve a bit deeper into the world of sea salt and begin to meander your way through the many different varieties—each with its own texture, color, and flavor, they get even more, um, interesting.

For the most part, sea salt is harvested in one of two ways: either via natural evaporation or through a process of boiling down seawater until all that's left is salt. When there is plenty of solar energy, salt water can be slowly (it can take up to five years!) evaporated by the sun, such as in France, where fleur de sel (French for "flower of salt") is harvested. In other parts of the world, where sun power is in short supply or less reliable, that previously mentioned boiling technique is employed, such as in the case of Maldon salt, a particular brand of flaked salt from the UK.

Regardless of which method is used, the faster the evaporation process (or, the higher the heat), the smaller the finished crystals will be. Conversely, a longer evaporation time and/or evaporation at lower temperatures allows for the formation of larger salt crystals and salt flakes. The way salt is raked, skimmed from the surface or allowed to settle to the bottom of a brine impacts whether it becomes a flat flake or crystal salt and—to be honest—going through the science of how all of *that* happens is a book in and of itself. Suffice it to say, quite a number of factors, ranging from climate to weather to the exact concentration of salt in a given body of water, dictate which kind of salt will be produced. What you want to know is which kind of sea salt to buy, how to store it, and how to use it, right? So, let's get to it!

Buying Sea Salt

I recommend you keep three types of sea salt around for your cooking, cleaning, and beauty uses. They are: an inexpensive everyday fine sea salt, an inexpensive everyday coarse sea salt, and at least one finishing salt, such as fleur de sel, Maldon salt or Cyprus flake, or something similar. The latter will, in all likelihood, lean a bit toward expensive, but remember that you'll be using it quite sparingly.

As for everyday salt, my recommendation is to taste several to help you decide which you like best. Once you've made a selection, stick with it! Always using the same salt will help provide consistency in your cooking, which will make your life easier. Trust me. I use French gray salt and kosher sea salt most often, as I find that they offer a kind of nuanced saltiness and flavor that appeals to me and their crystals dissolve easily in both baking and cooking, but neither is the only game in town. Remember, like wine or coffee or . . . well, olive oil, good salt carries the flavors and minerals of the place where it was harvested. And like wine or coffee or olive oil, what's more important than the pedigree of the product is whether it tastes good to *you*. Please do experiment to find something you love.

Finishing salts are the top shelf of sea salts and should be used only on a finished dish, sprinkled over food right before it's served. My first choice is fleur de sel, which is raked off the surface of salt marshes in France. The consistency is light and flaky, and the flavor is mild. I also use Maldon salt quite a bit. Both add a pleasing crunch and gentle saltiness to finished food. Other good finishing salts to consider: Trapani salt from Italy, Spanish flor de sal, Halen Môn from Wales, and Jacobsen, which is harvested in the Pacific Northwest.

How to Store Salt

Storing salt is pretty straightforward. Don't get it wet. That's all. Thanks for coming, everybody! Get home safe.

I'm kidding. Mostly. The truth is that storing salt is very uncomplicated. Its shelf life is indefinite, so you don't have to worry about your salt going bad. Beyond that, there are lots of convenient and stylish ways to store it on your countertop to make it accessible while you're cooking—from salt pigs (funny little ceramic vessels with wide openings that are specifically intended for storing salt) to fancy little wooden boxes or even a simple ramekin. I use a little red heart-shaped crock with a lid. It makes me happy. It doesn't much matter what you use,

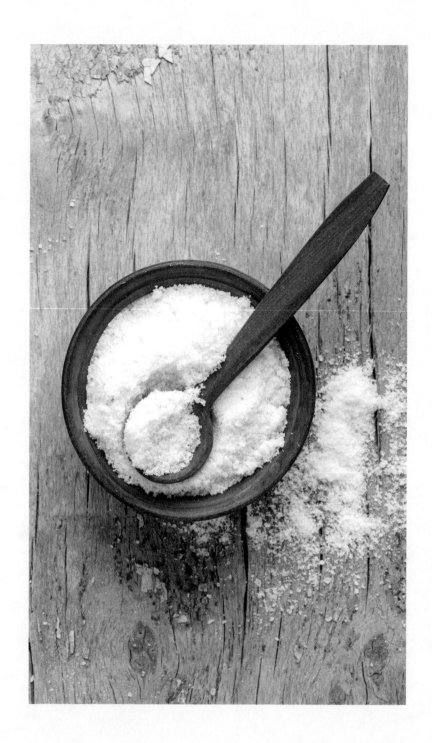

although I don't recommend storing salt in a metal container, as salt can eat away at metal over time, but find something large enough to hold a cup or so of salt at a time so you're not constantly refilling the container. Whatever you choose, make sure you are careful about cross-contaminating your salt. It helps to keep a spoon or small scoop nearby to avoid inadvertently sticking raw chicken–tainted fingers, for example, in your bowl of clean salt.

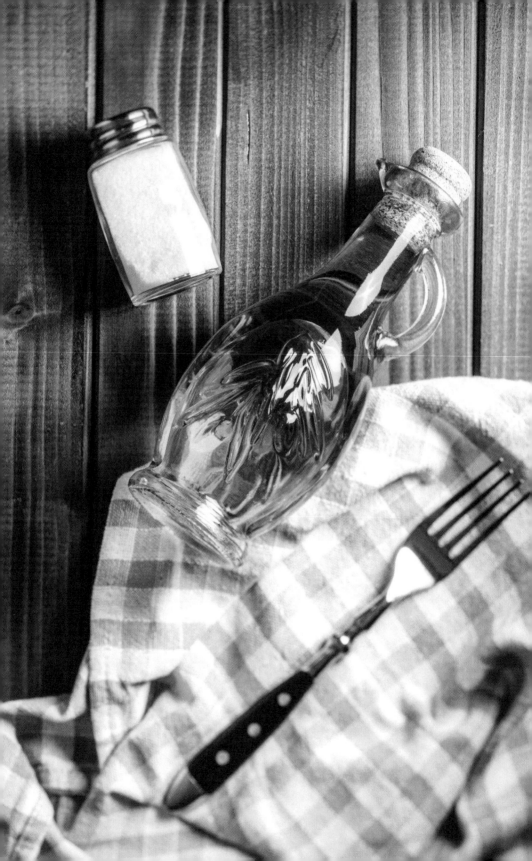

PART II

CLEVER WAYS TO USE OLIVE OIL AND SEA SALT AT HOME

DELICIOUS
RECIPES

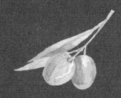

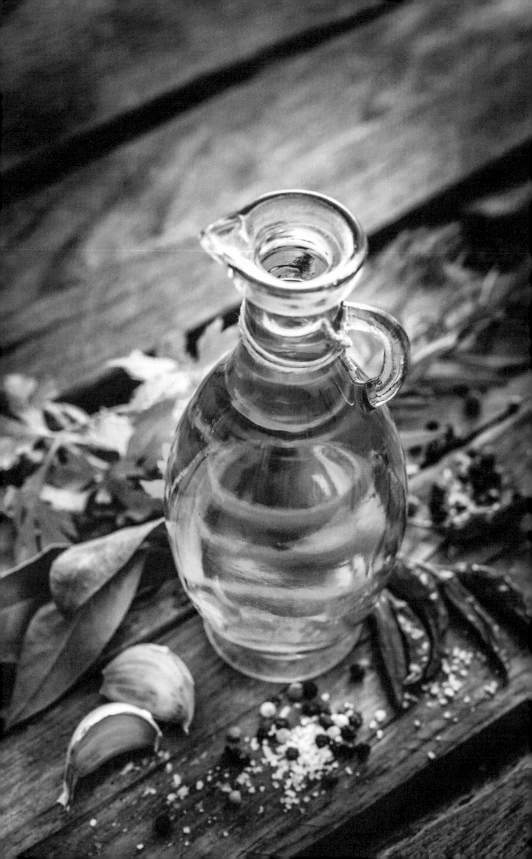

A Slew of Flavored Salts

Flavored salt—sometimes called finishing salt—is not something I had really considered making myself until I received some as a gift a number of years ago. It was smoked salt, a product new to me at the time. Intrigued but mildly unassured, I embarked on a little experiment, sprinkling a bit here and there, quickly realizing that it worked like a charm to add a pop of flavor to a dish without requiring a slew of spices. I sprinkled it on thick slices of tomatoes, on fish, and on steamed edamame for an extra layer of flavor. It brought depth to candied nuts, kicked up the smokiness of my baba ghanoush, and made something extra special out of simple buttered popcorn. The lightbulb went on and I *got* it!

My brain went into overdrive thinking about ways to play with other salt flavors in dishes, such as rosemary-salted potato chips, citrus salt on the rim of a margarita glass, and porcini mushroom salt sprinkled over fresh pasta, steak, or roasted potatoes. You see where I'm going here? Endless possibilities. Here are a few fantastic flavored salts for you to start playing with (or to give as gifts!).

Note: Each recipe makes about ½ cup of flavored salt. Use a flaky salt for the best texture and appearance. Try Maldon salt or fleur de sel.

VANILLA SALT

Subtle and versatile, vanilla salt is great on brownies and blondies, seared scallops, fresh lobster and . . . ready? Watermelon!

Makes about ½ cup flavored salt

½ cup sea salt
2 vanilla beans

1. Place the sea salt in a small bowl.

2. Using a sharp paring knife, trim the ends of the vanilla beans, split them lengthwise, and use the tip of the knife to scrape out the seeds and add them to the bowl of salt.

3. Rub the vanilla beans and salt together between your fingers until they're uniformly combined. Store in an airtight container at room temperature until ready to use.

4. Vanilla salt becomes more strongly flavored over time. It's best to wait at least 2 weeks before using it to give the vanilla time to infuse the salt.

LAVENDER SALT

I love lavender salt on chocolate desserts. It's also great on top of a slice of freshly baked, buttered bread and brings a lovely floral note to salads.

Makes about ½ cup flavored salt

½ cup sea salt
1 tablespoon culinary-grade dried lavender buds

1. Combine ¼ cup of the sea salt and the lavender in a spice grinder, clean coffee grinder, food processor, or mortar and pestle. Pulse until coarsely crushed.

2. Transfer to a small bowl and stir together with the remaining ¼ cup of sea salt.

3. Store in an airtight container at room temperature until ready to use.

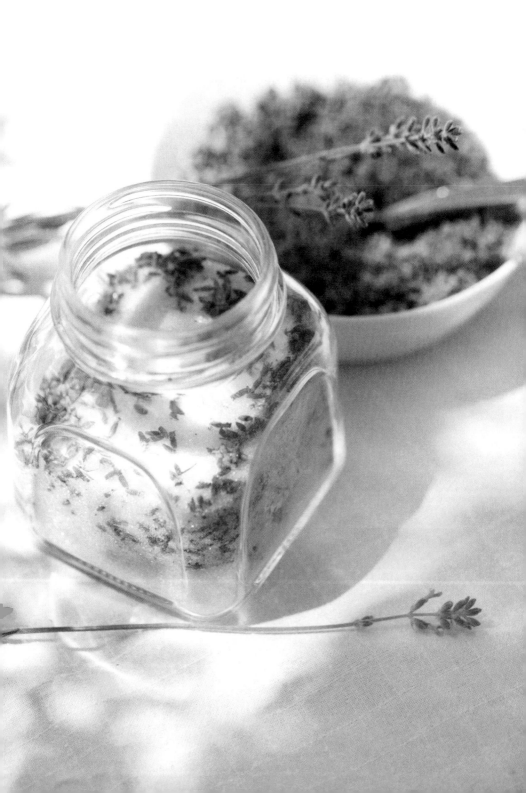

PORCINI SALT

Talk about an umami bomb! Use this stuff on steak, french fries, and risotto.

Makes about ½ cup flavored salt

¼ cup dried porcini mushrooms
½ cup sea salt

1. Combine the dried mushrooms and ¼ cup of the sea salt in a spice grinder, clean coffee grinder, food processor, or mortar and pestle and process until finely ground.

2. Transfer to a small bowl and stir together with the remaining sea salt.

3. Store in an airtight container at room temperature until ready to use.

SRIRACHA SALT

This red-hued finishing salt adds a fiery note to fried eggs, grilled chicken, salads, and even—believe it or not—vanilla ice cream.

Makes about ½ cup flavored salt

½ cup sea salt
1 tablespoon sriracha

1. Preheat your oven to 350°F. Line a baking sheet with parchment paper.

2. Combine the sea salt and sriracha in a small bowl, mix together, then spread over the prepared baking sheet.

3. Turn off the oven. Place pan inside and let it sit in the cooling oven for 3 to 4 hours, until fully dried out.

4. Store in an airtight container at room temperature until ready to use.

GOMASIO
(TOASTED SESAME SALT)

Gomasio is a traditional Japanese condiment and it's pretty fantastic on just about anything! Try it on salads, roasted vegetables, seared fish, and steamed rice. You can use white or black sesame seeds—or a mixture.

Makes about ½ cup flavored salt

½ cup white and/or black sesame seeds
1 teaspoon sea salt

1. Toast the sesame seeds in a dry skillet over medium heat, stirring often, until golden brown, about 5 minutes. Transfer to a food processor or spice grinder and let cool.

2. Add the sea salt to the sesame seeds and pulse until about half of the seeds are ground (there should still be some whole seeds), six to eight pulses.

3. Store in an airtight container at room temperature until ready to use.

ROSEMARY SALT

An excellent seasoning for eggs, potatoes, butternut squash, or chicken, this salt makes an especially lovely hostess or holiday gift.

Makes about ½ cup flavored salt

½ cup sea salt
1 to 2 teaspoons dried rosemary

1. Combine ¼ cup of the sea salt and the rosemary in a spice grinder, clean coffee grinder, food processor or mortar and pestle. Pulse until coarsely crushed.

2. Transfer to a small bowl and stir together with the remaining sea salt.

3. Store in an airtight container at room temperature until ready to use.

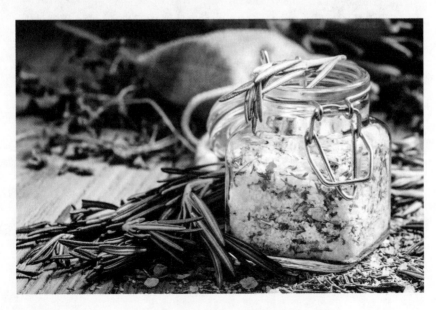

CITRUS SALT

Any kind of citrus works here—and a combination of, say, clementine and lime or lemon and grapefruit is really delicious. Try it sprinkled over curries or homemade salted caramels, as the finishing touch on steamed asparagus, or in cocktails. Obviously.

Makes about ½ cup flavored salt

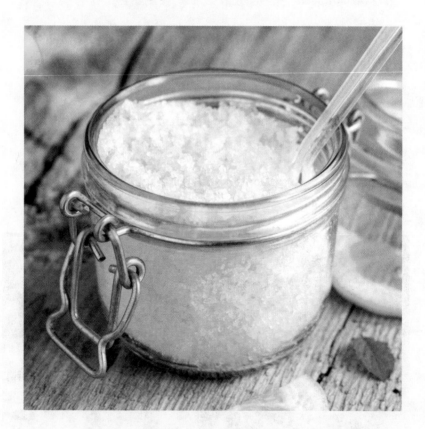

½ cup sea salt

1 tablespoon grated citrus zest

1. Preheat the oven to 225°F. Line a baking sheet with parchment paper.

2. Combine the salt and citrus in a small bowl. Rub the mixture together between your fingers until uniformly combined. Spread across the prepared baking sheet.

3. Bake for about an hour, or until the citrus is completely dried out. Remove from the oven and allow to cool a bit. At this point, you can pulse the citrus salt a few times in a food processor if you like, which is what I do. Or, you can enjoy it as is.

4. Store in an airtight jar at room temperature; will keep for a couple of months.

Vegetables and Sides

SAFFRON-ROASTED CAULIFLOWER WITH FLEUR DE SEL

Earthy cauliflower, perfumed with the subtly floral scent of saffron, doused in very good olive oil and blasted in a hot oven until deep, nutty brown, is a no-brainer of a vegetable dish. I just love the contrast here. On the one hand, there's saffron—quite the spice cabinet diva, with its hefty price tag (don't worry, you only need a pinch here) and its need to be treated *just so* to coax its inimitable flavor. On the other, there's cauliflower—humble and simple. Olive oil adds richness and depth, and a final sprinkling of flaky salt brings flavor and texture. You can serve it as a hearty side; as part of an assortment of tapas or meze; or tossed with pasta or farro, some feta, and a big handful of fresh parsley leaves for an easy weeknight dinner or packable lunch. Be sure to use your very best olive oil here—it makes a difference. And as for the salt, I suggest fleur de sel, but you can use any flaky sea salt you like. Maldon salt would be great, or try black lava salt, which would also add some visual interest to the dish.

Serves 4

¼ cup extra virgin olive oil

Pinch of saffron threads (about ¼ teaspoon)

1 large head cauliflower, cut into florets

¼ teaspoon coarse sea salt

Freshly ground black pepper

Fleur de sel for serving

Crushed red pepper flakes for serving (optional)

1. Preheat the oven to 450°F. Line a baking sheet with parchment.

2. Place 2 tablespoons of the olive oil and the saffron threads in a small saucepan or skillet. Heat gently over low heat until the olive oil is warm. Turn off the heat and allow it to steep for 5 to 10 minutes.

3. Combine the cauliflower florets, saffron oil, coarse salt, and pepper to taste in a large bowl and toss together. Spread the cauliflower on the prepared baking sheet and roast for 40 to 45 minutes, until golden brown, stirring halfway through.

4. When the cauliflower is done roasting, arrange it on a serving platter, drizzle it with the remaining 2 tablespoons of olive oil and sprinkle fleur de sel and crushed red pepper flakes (if using).

BLISTERED SHISHITO PEPPERS WITH GOMASIO

Shishito peppers are mild, little Japanese peppers that, when roasted or grilled, make a delicious, super addictive appetizer, side, or—my fave—cocktail accompaniment (it's five o'clock somewhere!). They are insanely easy to make—just toss them with olive oil and salt and either throw them under the broiler or into a hot cast-iron skillet for literally a few minutes, until they are a bit charred and blistered. You can finish them with anything from a squeeze of lemon to a drizzle of peanut sauce, but my favorite is with a sprinkling of gomasio (page 48) There's just something about the crunch against the soft and smoky peppers that is truly irresistible.

Serves 4 to 6 as a snack

12 ounces shishito peppers
1 tablespoon extra virgin olive oil
Coarse sea salt
Gomasio (page 48; optional)

1. Heat a large, ovenproof skillet under the broiler or (need not be ovenproof) on the stovetop over high heat.

2. Place the peppers in a bowl. Drizzle them with 1 table-spoon of the olive oil and a healthy sprinkle of coarse salt. Toss to coat.

3. Transfer the peppers to the skillet under the broiler or on the stovetop (lower the heat to medium-high) and cook without disturbing them for 1 to 2 minutes, until they begin to char on the bottom. Continue to cook, stirring every minute or two, until the peppers are blistered and darkened all over, about 5 minutes total.

4. Transfer the peppers to a plate and sprinkle with gomasio or more coarse salt. Serve immediately.

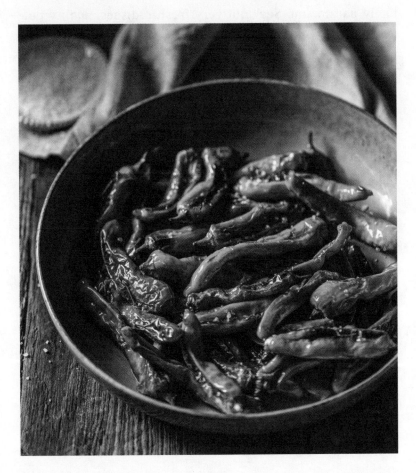

FRENCH-STYLE RADISHES WITH BUTTER AND SEA SALT

This delicious, well-loved way of serving radishes is *très Français* and truly couldn't be simpler. It's hardly a recipe at all, really—just radishes, spread with some butter and sprinkled with salt. But here's the thing: this is one of those instances where the quality of the ingredients you choose is absolutely paramount. Seek out very fresh radishes, quality butter (European-style butter would be most welcome here), and a good, flaky salt. It's the perfect balance of spicy and sweet, with the radish's bite toned down by the salt and its heat mellowed by the creamy butter. Although I'm often one to err on the side of keeping things simple, you have my full support should you decide to shake things up a bit and swap out the flaked salt here for a flavored one, such as lavender (page 44), vanilla (page 43), or citrus (page 50). *Bon appétit!*

Serves 4 to 6 as an hors d'oeuvre

1 bunch radishes, rinsed and dried

3 tablespoons unsalted butter, at room temperature

1 tablespoon flaky sea salt or table salt

1. While keeping most of the stems intact, halve the radishes vertically from the root to tip.

2. Serve the radishes with the butter and a bowl of flaky sea salt or table salt.

SAUERKRAUT

Sauerkraut—probably best known as a topping for hot dogs and sandwiches (well, hello there, Reuben!)—is surprisingly easy to make at home. All you need to get your probiotic party started is a head of cabbage and some salt. Oh, and about a week's time. Here's the quick lowdown on how this whole naturally fermented food thing works: *Lactobacillus* bacteria is present pretty much everywhere—on our body, on the surface of the cabbage here and, in fact, on all fruits and vegetables. They're generally considered "friendly" bacteria, meaning they're not harmful to us.

During sauerkraut fermentation, when shredded cabbage is submerged in a salty brine, the *Lactobacillus* begin to convert naturally occurring sugars into lactic acid, which is a natural preservative that inhibits the growth of harmful bacteria. It is also what makes naturally fermented things, such as pickles, kimchi, yogurt, and, yes, sauerkraut, taste sour. This process, called lacto-fermentation, has been used for eons; aside from extending the shelf life of the cabbage, it also transforms it into something tasty and healthy, because sauerkraut is chock-full of gut-friendly probiotics. With minimal effort, all of two ingredients, and a bit of patience, you can make your very own crunchy, delicious sauerkraut at home.

Makes about 1 quart sauerkraut

Continued

1 medium head green cabbage (about 3 pounds), trimmed, cored, and shredded

2 tablespoons Maldon salt or other coarse sea salt

1. Place the shredded cabbage in a large bowl and sprinkle the Maldon salt over the top.

2. Using your hands, begin working the salt into the cabbage by massaging and squeezing it. Continue to knead the cabbage for 5 to 10 minutes, until it becomes very watery and limp.

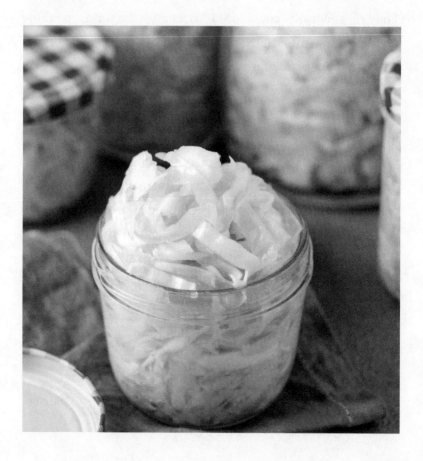

3. Transfer the seasoned cabbage to a clean 1-quart mason jar, reserving the liquid, and tamp down the cabbage to pack it into the jar. A wooden spoon works well for this.

4. Pour the reserved liquid released by the cabbage into the jar.

5. Once all the cabbage is packed into the mason jar, slip a fermentation weight, if you have one, into the mouth of the jar, or use a small jelly jar filled with clean stones or marbles to weigh down the cabbage. This will keep the cabbage submerged beneath its liquid.

6. Top the jar with a fermentation lid or a piece of cloth secured with a rubber band and leave it at room temperature, away from direct sunlight, to ferment for 5 to 7 days.

7. Check the sauerkraut daily to make sure it remains submerged. If not, press down on it to keep it under the liquid. Start tasting it after 5 days—when the sauerkraut tastes good to you, remove the weight, screw on a lid, and refrigerate it for up to 6 months.

Note: Don't worry about any bubbles you might see coming through the cabbage, or even foam on the top. These are all signs of healthy, happy fermentation. Mold, on the other hand— anything green, black, red, or pink, or in raised fuzzy spots—is not a welcome party guest and should be scraped off before refrigerating.

PRESERVED LEMONS

"When life gives you lemons . . ." oh, you know the rest. Okay, sure, when life gives you lemons, you *could* make lemonade, but you can also make preserved lemons—a fermented condiment commonly used in North African and Middle Eastern cuisine—which are, in my opinion, infinitely more interesting and incredibly easy to make. Originally conceived as a way to eat lemons in the off-season, preserved lemons bring a flavor and quality to a dish that regular lemons cannot—they're citrusy and floral, yet somehow also savory. The salt tempers the intensity of regular lemons and smooths out their bitterness, and time softens the rind, making it easy to chop and toss into an array of Middle Eastern recipes. But please don't stop there, because the salty, sweet-and-sour burst of flavor that preserved lemons impart is a beautiful addition to pasta, salads, pan sauces, and even Bloody Marys.

This recipe makes a large batch, which is great news, because they keep for a really long time in the fridge. (Ahem, they're preserved, no?) How long? I'm going to be conservative here and say that you should use them within six months, but I've kept them in my fridge closer to a year and I'm literally still here to tell the tale. So, no rush. They also make a lovely gift, so consider packing them into smaller jars and/or doubling or tripling the recipe. Just be sure to use very clean jars; I recommend sterilizing them in boiling water for 15 minutes and drying them well before proceeding with the recipe.

Makes 1 quart preserved lemons

8 to 10 lemons, scrubbed well to remove dirt and impurities

Sea salt

1. Cut each lemon into quarters lengthwise, without slicing through the base.

2. Add about 2 tablespoons of sea salt to the bottom of the jar and pack the lemons into the jar, pressing on them to release their juice. Add more salt after each layer of lemons. Fill the jar, but leave about an inch of headroom.

3. Add 2 more tablespoons of salt to the top. Seal the jar.

4. Leave the jar on the counter for 2 to 3 days, shaking it once a day to distribute the salt and liquids.

5. Move the jar to the refrigerator and allow it to cure for about 3 weeks, or until the rinds have softened.

6. To use, rinse the lemons thoroughly to remove excess salt and discard the seeds, then use as you like.

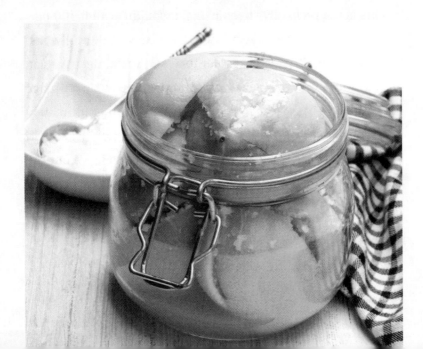

KIMCHI

One of our favorite family outings is a weekend trip to our local Asian supermarket. It's full of exciting, delicious, and otherwise hard-to-find ingredients. My husband loves to go hunting in the snack aisle, my kids like to check out the samples, and I get lost in the produce aisle, where I can find treasures such as shiso leaves, long beans, and galangal. Perhaps we're just a very easily entertained bunch of food nerds, but it really is fun for the whole family. One item on our perpetual must-buy list *used to* be kimchi, which we would choose from a dizzying array. And by that I mean there is an entire wall dedicated to kimchi—cabbage, cucumber, pumpkin . . . dozens and dozens of brands, types, and sizes. After one of our weekend excursions, I texted a photo of our impressive haul to my brother—also a kimchi fan—to which he responded, "I've been making my own kimchi." *Wait, what?* He insisted it was easy and much, much less expensive. I decided to give it a try.

This is the recipe I've been using. I wouldn't call it 100 percent authentic, but it is very good, very easy, and totally customizable to suit your heat tolerance and taste. Because you already know how to make sauerkraut (if not, give it a try [page 57]), this will be a piece of (powerful smelling, but ultimately very delicious) cake, as it's a similar fermentation process. If you're vegetarian or allergic to fish, feel free to leave out the fish sauce or shrimp paste. The finished product will still be wonderfully salty, sour, and crunchy.

Makes 1 quart kimchi

1 head napa cabbage (about 2 pounds), cut into 2-by-1-inch rectangles

2 tablespoons coarse sea salt

2 teaspoons minced garlic

1 teaspoon grated fresh ginger

2 tablespoons Asian fish sauce or shrimp paste (optional)

1 teaspoon sugar

3 tablespoons gochugaru (Korean chile pepper flakes)—more or less to taste

4 scallions, green parts only, cut into 2-inch pieces

1 small yellow onion, thinly sliced

Continued

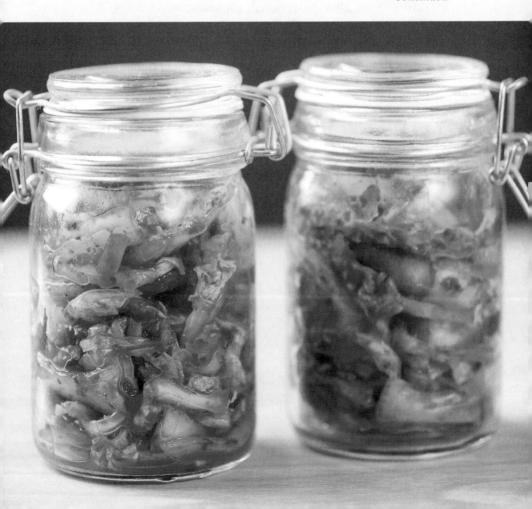

1. Place the cabbage in a large bowl and sprinkle with the coarse salt. Using your hands, massage the salt into the cabbage until it starts to soften a bit. Set aside for about 50 minutes.

2. Drain the liquid and rinse the cabbage to remove the salt. Drain the cabbage in a colander for 10 to 15 minutes.

3. Meanwhile, mix together the garlic, ginger, fish sauce (if using), and sugar in a small bowl until you achieve a paste. Stir in the gochugaru, using about 1 tablespoon if you like it mild and up to 5 tablespoons for crazy spicy (I like about 2½ tablespoons); set aside.

4. Combine the scallions, yellow onions, seasoning paste, and cabbage in a large bowl. Mix until the seasoning paste is distributed evenly.

5. Pack the mixture tightly into a very clean 1-quart mason jar or another glass container, pressing down as you fill it. Seal the jar and place a plate or bowl underneath to catch any overflow of liquid.

6. Let the jar stand at cool room temperature, away from direct sunlight, for 3 to 5 days, tasting it after day 3. When the kimchi is ripe enough for your liking, transfer the jar to the refrigerator. Consume within 6 months to a year.

Note: You can check to see how your fermentation is coming along by opening the lid and taking a peek; you should see some bubbling juices (but no mold!) and taste the tanginess of the freshly pickled cabbage.

GREEK-STYLE BOILED GREENS (HORTA)

Horta is Greek for "weeds"—it's a blanket term for any sort of edible wild greens, such as dandelion, amaranth, mustard, and chicory. In Greece, horta is usually boiled, dressed simply with olive oil and lemon, as here, and some would argue that it's one of the healthiest foods on earth. Sound hyperbolic? Well, the Greek island of Ikaria, where more than 150 different varieties of edible greens grow, has been documented to have one of the highest concentrations in the world of people living more than 100 years. And Ikarians eat horta pretty much every day. So, you do the math! Leftover greens are great topped with a fried egg (see page 114 for the perfect fried egg).

Serves 4

8 cups leafy greens and/or wild herbs (chicory, kale, dandelion, escarole, etc.), cleaned to remove dirt and sand

¼ cup extra virgin olive oil

3 tablespoons fresh lemon juice

Sea salt

1. Fill a large stockpot with salted water and bring to a boil. Add the greens to the pot and cook until the stalks are fork-tender. Their cooking time will vary depending on the type of greens you choose—2 to 3 minutes for spinach and other delicate greens, but more like 15 to 20 minutes for a hardier variety like dandelion greens or collards.

2. Drain the greens and dress with the olive oil, lemon juice, and sea salt to taste. Serve warm or at room temperature.

OLIVE OIL MASHED POTATOES

Buttery, creamy mashed potatoes made with *all* the dairy is an indisputably delicious food. There's a reason many a Thanksgiving just can't happen without them. I, for the most part, am not in favor of messing with a classic recipe like that. Not when it's so nearly perfect. That said, potatoes mashed with olive oil are not merely "dairy-free" mashed potatoes or vegan mashed potatoes (although both happen to be true)—they are a distinct food entirely and they, too, are indisputably delicious.

While they're definitely creamy, these potatoes are more potato-y than buttery, heavy cream–laden mashed potatoes. Absent the richness of the traditional version, these give way for the full flavor of the potatoes and the olive oil shines through. A sprinkling of good Parmesan added to the dish would not be frowned upon, nor would the addition of roasted garlic be discouraged, but a final drizzle of fruity olive oil and a sprinkling of flaky salt is really all you need.

Serves 4

2½ pounds Yukon Gold potatoes, peeled and roughly chopped

1 tablespoon flaky sea salt

Freshly ground black pepper

⅓ cup extra virgin olive oil, plus more for serving

1. Put the potatoes in a large saucepan, cover with cool water, and add a pinch of sea salt. Bring the water to a boil, lower the heat to a simmer, and cook for 12 to 15 minutes, until they're easy to pierce with a fork.

2. Drain the potatoes, then transfer them to a large bowl and immediately pass them through a ricer or food mill or mash them with a potato masher or the back of a wooden spoon. Stir in the flaky salt and olive oil.

3. Serve immediately, sprinkled with more flaky salt and a drizzle of oil.

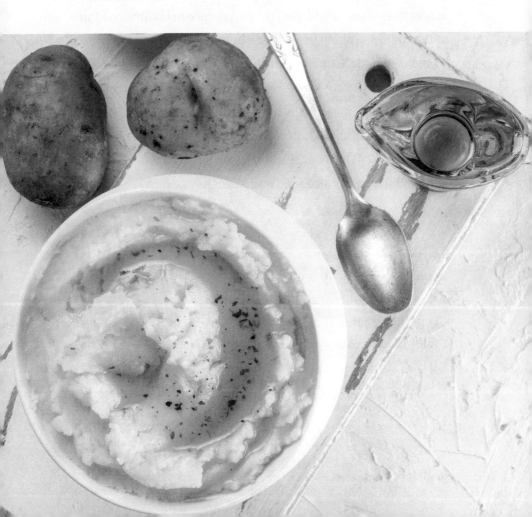

BRAISED LEEKS

Leeks always make me think of Julia Child. As a kid (long before the Food Network existed), when I was home sick from school, I'd almost always spend part of my convalescence watching a marathon of cooking shows on PBS. I'd happily watch hours of *The Frugal Gourmet*, *Yan Can Cook*, *The Galloping Gourmet*, *Ciao Italia*, *Everyday Cooking with Jacques Pépin* . . . all of them. And Julia, of course. I remember watching her cook with leeks and thinking they were oh so sophisticated and fancy, which is funny, because they're really considered quite the humble veg in most other parts of the world. But, they were rare in the United States at the time, definitely not a staple in my house growing up, and, as such, I found them quite intimidating for a very long time.

Now, I appreciate leeks for their mellow, sweet flavor. This dish, very much inspired by a recipe Julia cooked on-air at some point in my childhood, is meltingly delicious. It's a fabulous accompaniment to roast chicken (page 98). And I love using the leftovers in eggs or as a sandwich filling.

Serves 4

6 large leeks
½ cup extra virgin olive oil
Sea salt and freshly ground black pepper
1 cup sliced shallots
1 tablespoon fresh thyme leaves, or 1 teaspoon dried
1½ cups chicken stock, vegetable stock, or water
½ cup dry white wine

1. Preheat the oven to 400°F.

2. Trim the roots, remove the outer leaves from the leeks, and cut off the dark green ends. Cut the leeks in half lengthwise and submerge in a large bowl of cold water, shaking well to dislodge any dirt, then leave them alone for a minute or two. Remove from the water, then repeat the process with clean water until no dirt or sand remains. Pat the leeks dry with paper towels.

3. Heat ¼ cup of the olive oil in a large skillet over medium heat. Add the leeks to the pan and arrange them, cut side down, in a single layer. (You may need to cook them in batches.) Cook until softened and lightly golden, 3 to 4 minutes. Turn the leeks and cook on the other side until softened, for 3 minutes. Season with salt and pepper.

4. Transfer the leeks to a large gratin or casserole dish, arranging them cut side up. Set aside.

5. Heat ¼ cup of the olive oil to the same skillet you used for the leeks, over medium heat. Add the shallots, thyme, ¼ teaspoon of sea salt, and a pinch of pepper. Cook just until the shallots begin to brown at the edges, about 5 minutes. Add the stock and wine, stirring to deglaze pan. Cook for 1 minute.

6. Pour the shallot mixture over the leeks. Cover the baking dish with a piece of parchment cut to fit or with a lid. Bake until the leeks are tender when pierced with a knife, about 30 minutes.

MASSAGED BRUSSELS SPROUT SALAD WITH OLIVE OIL, LEMON, AND PECORINO

Shaving raw Brussels sprouts is a popular and lovely way to serve these sturdy little vegetables. Shredded whisper-thin, it's a dish that sits somewhere between slaw and salad—hearty and satisfying, yet light. The one problem I've found with treating Brussels sprouts in this manner, however, is that they aren't exactly the most tender vegetables around and they can sometimes end up being a lot of work to chew! I'll save my workouts for the gym, thank you very much, and instead add one extra step to the process to ensure they're just the right level of crunch: massaging them with salt. It's a technique I borrowed from both a massaged kale salad recipe I make a few times a week for my family, and from the first step in making sauerkraut (page 57).

Tossing raw Brussels sprouts with salt and then kneading and massaging them with your hands wilts them via our old friend osmosis as well as simply the brute force of crushing them a bit manually. The rest is simple—some very good extra virgin olive oil, fragrant lemon, and salty pecorino (or, really, any hard and salty cheese you like). I do recommend using a mandoline to shred the sprouts, if you have one, as you'll achieve the most delicate texture that way, but you can certainly use a sharp knife or even the slicing blade on your food processor, if you prefer.

Serves 4

1½ pounds Brussels sprouts, trimmed and shredded
    or thinly sliced

½ teaspoon coarse sea salt, plus more to taste

3 tablespoons extra virgin olive oil

2 to 3 tablespoons fresh lemon juice

¼ cup fresh herbs, such as chives, parsley, or thyme
    (or a mixture), minced

2 ounces pecorino or another hard, salty, aged cheese, shaved
    (Parmesan, ricotta salata, etc.)

1. Toss the shredded Brussels sprouts with the coarse salt in
   a medium bowl. Knead and squeeze the sprouts, softening
   them and perhaps releasing a bit of their liquid (depending
   on the age and water content of your sprouts), about 1 minute. Set aside for 10 minutes.

2. Drain out any liquid that has accumulated under the Brussels sprouts. Toss gently with the olive oil, lemon juice, and
   herbs. Add the cheese and toss again.

CHERRY TOMATO CONFIT

What's confit? I'm so glad you asked! *Confit* ("kon-FEE") is a French word that refers to a very old, but still-used, method of food preservation whereby food (originally meat, such as duck, goose, or pork) is salted and slowly cooked in (its own) fat. Once upon a time, in the days before refrigeration, this cooking method was utilized out of necessity to extend the shelf life of perishable foods. As it turns out, it also makes food—not

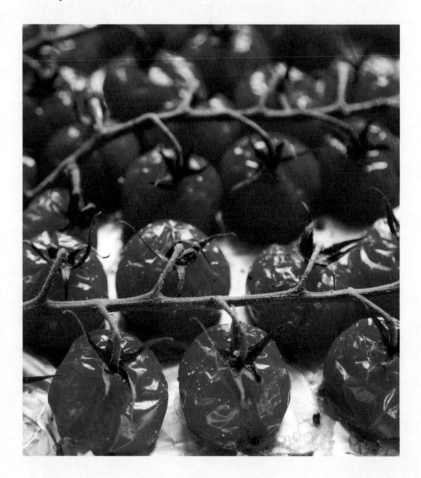

just meat, but vegetables, too—taste incredibly delicious and luxurious in flavor and texture, which is likely why it didn't disappear with the advent of refrigeration.

Cherry tomatoes prepared as confit become soft, sweet, and meltingly smooth. The recipe does take a while, but I promise that it is worth it. Plus, you can spend that time dreaming up all the many ways in which you'll eat these beauties: spread on toast, as an accompaniment to cheese and crackers, tossed with pasta, layered on pizza, smeared on meat or fish . . . And the infused oil is perfect for dipping bread or stirring into a vinaigrette.

Makes about 1 quart confit

2 pints cherry tomatoes

1½ cups extra virgin olive oil, or as needed

4 garlic cloves, peeled and smashed

1 teaspoon coarse sea salt

1. Preheat the oven to 225°F.

2. Place the tomatoes in a baking dish large enough to hold them in a single layer. Pour the oil over the tomatoes and add the garlic and coarse salt. Bake, uncovered, until the tomatoes are swollen and the skins are wrinkled, about 3 hours.

3. Remove from the oven and allow to cool. Transfer the confit, including the olive oil and garlic, into a 1-quart jar or other airtight container. Refrigerate for up to 1 month.

WHITE BEAN MASH WITH HERB OIL

Even though I do most of the cooking, meal planning, and grocery shopping in our house, my husband is in charge of keeping track of our pantry staples, managing our inventory of dried pasta, rice, tuna, crushed tomatoes, canned beverages, and snack foods. Canned beans are part of his domain and he makes sure we always have a few different varieties on hand, which has saved me on more than one occasion as I've scrambled to get dinner on the table.

Super versatile cannellini beans are a favorite around here, with their mild flavor and intrinsic creaminess. Here, they're mashed and adorned with a vibrant herb oil that comes together easily in a blender or food processor—I suggest using chives, parsley, and basil, but you can absolutely use whatever you have on hand. It's a dish that is easy enough to round out a mad dash weeknight dinner (and may even qualify as a main dish if you pair it with a salad and some bread), but is pretty enough to serve alongside roast chicken, meat, or fish.

Serves 4

HERB OIL

½ cup roughly chopped fresh chives

½ cup fresh parsley leaves and stems

½ cup fresh basil leaves

½ cup extra virgin olive oil

Squeeze of lemon juice

Coarse sea salt

BEANS

2 tablespoons olive oil

2 garlic cloves, crushed

Two 15-ounce cans cannellini beans, drained and rinsed

Sea salt and freshly ground black pepper

½ cup chicken stock, vegetable stock, or water

Flaky sea salt for serving

1. Prepare the herb oil: Combine the herbs in a food processor or high-speed blender and pulse until finely chopped.

2. Add the olive oil and pulse again until the mixture is completely emulsified. Add the lemon juice and pulse to combine. Transfer to a small bowl, add coarse sea salt to taste, and set aside.

3. Prepare the beans: Heat the 2 tablespoons of olive oil in a large skillet over medium-low heat. Add the garlic and cook until fragrant, about 1 minute. Add the beans and warm through, stirring and smashing with a wooden spoon or spatula until most of the beans have become a

Continued

rough puree. You should have a few intact beans here and there, but you're mostly looking for a rough sort of mush. Season with salt and pepper.

4. Add the stock or water and bring the mixture to a gentle simmer. Cook for 2 to 3 minutes, until the beans become creamy and slightly thickened.

5. Transfer the beans to a serving bowl and drizzle or swirl the herb oil on top. Season with flaky salt. Serve warm.

Mains

OLIVE OIL-POACHED FISH WITH GARLIC AND HERBS

Here it is, folks, the secret to cooking flawless fish: olive oil poaching. Using a classic French technique as the foundation (poaching, which means cooking something slowly in flavorful liquid), this riff involves submerging a piece of fish in a bath of warm, herb-scented olive oil and then cooking it in the oven at a low temperature to succulent perfection. Almost impossible to overcook, the fish here emerges from its spa vacation tender and silky and not—as you might suspect—even the least bit greasy.

The method requires a fair amount of oil, so please don't use the most expensive, super premium olive oil you have on the shelf for this. On the other hand, please don't use absolute garbagio, either. Pick an oil that sits somewhere in the middle—and make sure it tastes good to you!

As far as choosing fish, oil poaching works especially well with firm, meaty fish, such as tuna, salmon, halibut, and snapper. But—really—any other type, from tilapia to Dover sole, and even peeled shrimp or scallops, will work just fine. And as for the aromatics, here I suggest garlic, lemon, fresh thyme, and dill because they are classic flavors, but I highly recommend giving other flavor combinations a try, too—fennel and orange, saffron, ginger, and sesame . . . they're all so good!

Serves 4

Continued

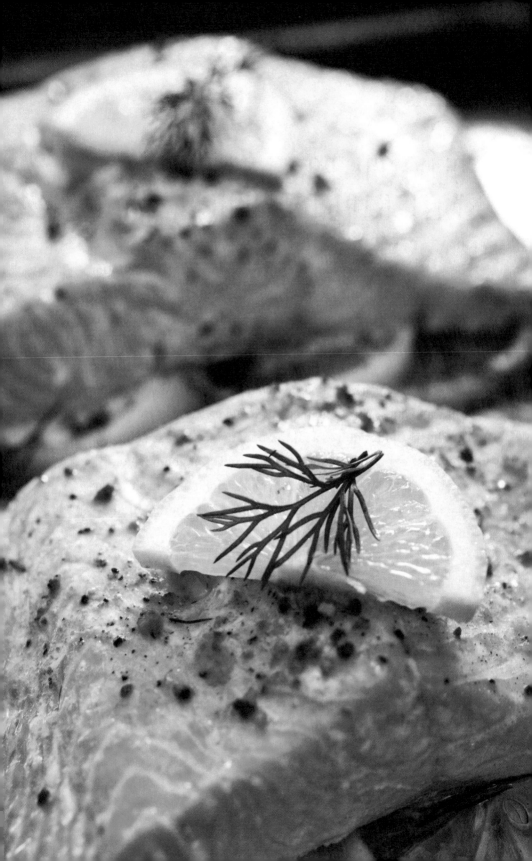

1½ to 2 pounds skin-on firm fish, such as salmon, mahi-mahi, swordfish, or halibut—fillets cut into 4 pieces or steaks

Kosher salt and freshly ground black pepper

Extra virgin olive oil, for poaching

1 lemon, sliced into ¼-inch rounds

2 garlic cloves, peeled and halved

4 sprigs fresh thyme

2 sprigs fresh dill

1. Preheat your oven to 275°F.

2. Generously season the fish with kosher salt. Coat the bottom of a 3- to 4-quart baking pan or casserole dish (or another ovenproof vessel that will hold them snugly) with oil, then add the fish, skin side down. Nestle the lemon slices, garlic, and herb sprigs evenly among the pieces of fish. Add just enough oil to fully submerge the fish (about 1 cup).

3. Place the baking dish in the oven and allow the fish to cook until it is fairly firm and mostly opaque—this can take anywhere from 15 to 30 minutes, depending on thickness and type of fish you're using. Remove with a fish spatula or slotted spoon, allowing excess oil to drip back into the pot.

Note: Don't get rid of that oil! It's delicious and totally worth saving at least some of it. Serve the fish with crusty bread and use the reserved poaching oil for dipping. Or let it cool and stir some of the oil into a simple vinaigrette for any salad you may be serving alongside. And *definitely* drizzle at least a little bit of that flavorful oil on top of the fish when you bring it to the table! You can also save the oil and use it one or two more times to poach fish again. Just cover and refrigerate between uses.

SALT-BAKED FISH

Salt-baked fish is pretty much what it sounds like: a whole fish encrusted in salt and baked in the oven. The first time I tasted it was as a dinner guest while visiting friends in Spain. Our host (an expat from England, not a Spaniard, but a fantastic cook!) presented the whole baked fish encased in a minor mountain of salt and dramatically cracked it open tableside, revealing a succulent dish, with pure, clean ocean flavor and not a trace of saltiness. Served with homemade saffron aioli and roasted potatoes, the meal was utterly simple and yet one of the most memorable of my life. As it turns out, save for the perfect Spanish summer air and easy-breezy vacation feel, re-creating that fish experience at home is incredibly easy to do and virtually impossible to overcook, as the salt crust traps the moisture and ensures the fish comes out perfectly.

Have your fishmonger clean and scale the fish for you—any lean, white, flaky fish will do, including sea bass, flounder, red snapper, rockfish, or tilapia. Once cooked, fillet the fish and serve simply with your very best extra virgin olive oil, lemon wedges, and whatever sauce speaks to you: gremolata, pesto, saffron aioli, or even just a shower of minced fresh parsley.

Serves 4

2 whole fish (1½ to 2 pounds each) or 1 whole fish
   (about 3 pounds), cleaned and scaled
Handful of fresh herbs
1 lemon, thinly sliced
Drizzle of olive oil
6 cups coarse sea salt or kosher salt
2 large egg whites

1. Preheat the oven to 400°F.

2. Pat the fish dry inside and out with paper towels. Stuff
   each fish cavity with half of the herbs and lemon. Very
   lightly oil the entire outside of the fish with olive oil.

3. Combine the salt and egg whites in a medium bowl, mixing the ingredients together with your hands or a wooden
   spoon. Add a bit of water to the mixture until it resembles
   wet sand.

4. On a sheet pan, create a ¼-inch-thick layer of the salt mixture that's approximately the size of the two (or single
   large) fish. Lay the fish on the bed of salt and mound the
   remaining salt mixture around each fish, about ¼ inch
   thick, pressing and molding to create a tight seal.

5. Bake for 30 minutes, then remove from the oven and allow
   to rest for 10 minutes. Carefully crack and then break off
   the salt crust and fillet the fish inside. Serve immediately.

SCALLOPS WITH VANILLA SALT

I love scallops. They require very little preparation; they cook in about five minutes; they're quite versatile and work with lots of quick dinner bases, such as pasta, rice, and couscous; and with nothing more than a screaming hot pan and liberal seasoning, they make a showstopper of a main dish for a special occasion or an ordinary Tuesday night. And—bonus—scallops are almost always a sustainable seafood choice, grown and harvested with little environmental impact. Here, sea scallops are adorned with a dusting of vanilla salt (page 43), which takes them to a whole new level. Vanilla heightens the natural sweetness of scallops, and the crunch of the coarse salt provides a lovely textural contrast to their tender flesh.

Serves 4

1 to 1½ pounds dry sea scallops
Kosher salt
1 tablespoon vegetable oil
Vanilla Salt (page 43)
Freshly ground black pepper

1. Season the scallops on both sides with about ½ teaspoon of kosher salt. Place them on a paper towel–lined plate, cover them with another layer of paper towels, and refrigerate for 15 to 30 minutes.

2. Remove from the fridge and pat dry. Heat the vegetable oil in a large skillet over high heat until shimmering. Add the scallops, being careful not to crowd the pan, and sear them for 1 to 2 minutes per side, until they are nicely browned and caramelized. They will release from the pan easily once they're ready, and they should still be ever so slightly wobbly in the middle—they will continue to cook off the heat. Transfer the scallops to a paper towel–lined plate to drain.

3. Serve immediately, sprinkled with vanilla salt and pepper.

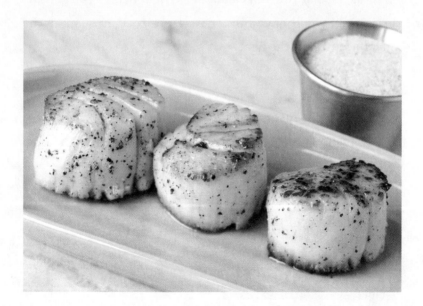

CHINESE SALT AND PEPPER SHRIMP

Here's one of those dishes that will sometimes stupefy me with its unexpected deliciousness, as the ingredient list is so short! I don't know why I'm surprised, though, as it's an undisputed fact that a great many ingredients does not necessarily equate to great food. In fact, some of the most sublime meals one can eat call for only a handful of top-notch ingredients (think: cacio e pepe or simple roast chicken). This shrimp makes one of those meals, for sure. Shrimp, salt, and two kinds of pepper take a quick dip in hot oil, are then adorned with fresh cilantro, and end up as a crunchy, salty, spicy, herbaceous, and floral treat that is ready in about 15 minutes, tops. If you start a pot of rice just before you get this dish going, you'll have dinner ready to rock as soon as the shrimp comes off the heat.

Serves 4

1½ pounds large shrimp, cleaned, tail-on

3 tablespoons cornstarch

1 teaspoon freshly ground black pepper

1½ teaspoons coarse sea salt

1 cup vegetable oil

1 teaspoon freshly ground Sichuan peppercorns

1 hot chile, such as jalapeño or serrano, thinly sliced, seeds removed if desired (optional)

½ cup fresh cilantro leaves

1. Pat the shrimp dry. Combine the cornstarch, black pepper, and ¾ teaspoon of the coarse salt in a large bowl; add the shrimp and toss to coat.

2. Heat the oil in a large skillet or wok over medium-high heat, until shimmering. Working in batches, fry the shrimp until golden, crisp, and cooked through, about 1 minute per side. Transfer to a paper towel–lined plate to drain, then toss in a medium bowl with the Sichuan peppercorns and remaining ¾ teaspoon of coarse salt. Add the chile and cilantro to the bowl and toss again.

Note: Sichuan peppercorns—all at once spicy, citrusy, and floral—are a dark-colored spice that produces a sort of tingly, almost numbing sensation on your tongue (in a good way!). They're worth seeking out and, I'm afraid, their unique flavor can't really be replaced with anything else. That said, this dish will still be delicious if you have to use something like red pepper flakes or pink peppercorns in place of the Sichuan peppercorns—it just won't be the same.

GRAVLAX

In my house, there is a very easy answer to the question "What is your family's favorite breakfast?" Bagels with lox and cream cheese, of course! My kids especially love it and can decimate an unfathomable quantity of lox in a sitting. But satisfying the quantity of lox my kids want to eat would be pretty expensive. So, from time to time I make my own. Well, sort of.

Did you know that lox isn't really lox? What I mean is that the stuff we typically eat with our bagels and call "lox" is actually smoked salmon. *Real* lox is salmon that's been packed in a massive amount of salt and left to cure for weeks. It's super salty and—in my opinion—just shy of edible. Gravlax, on the other hand, is a traditional Nordic dish of salmon that's been cured with salt and sugar and infused with the flavor of a variety of aromatics. It's clearly not the same as *smoked* salmon, but it's really delicious on a bagel (or served as an hors d'oeuvre alongside a glass of Champagne—you're welcome) and—best of all—it's a totally doable kitchen project that, yes, takes a bit of time but requires very little effort. One very important thing to note is that you should buy the absolute best-quality, freshest fish you can get your hands on. I recommend asking for sushi-grade salmon. Not only will it turn out a fantastic finished product, but it will have a longer shelf life than a lesser-quality piece of fish.

Makes about 1 pound gravlax

3 tablespoons kosher or coarse sea salt

¼ cup dark brown sugar

1 tablespoon freshly ground black pepper

1 pound skin-on, sushi-grade salmon fillet
(pin bones removed by fishmonger)

1 large bunch dill, chopped

1. Toss together the kosher salt, sugar, and pepper in a small bowl, mixing until thoroughly combined.

2. Lay the salmon, skin side down, in a glass or stainless steel baking dish. Sprinkle the salt mixture evenly over the salmon until completely covered. Cover the salt mixture with the chopped dill.

Continued

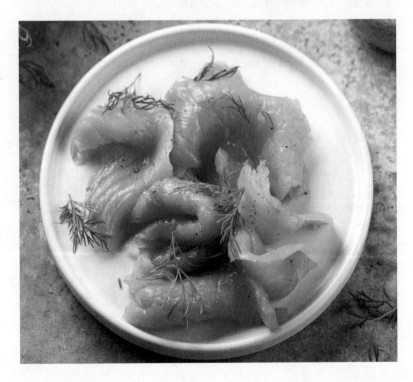

3. Cover the salmon with plastic wrap or a piece of parchment paper, then top with a weight (such as a smaller baking dish or plate with cans of beans on top). Refrigerate for 5 days.

4. Each day, remove the weight, flip the wrapped fish, and replace the weight, which will keep your fish more level and will help it slice more easily and evenly.

5. Remove salmon from the cure, which will likely have become liquefied at this point, brushing off the dill with a paper towel. You may also rinse the salmon with water if you'd like to remove even more of the salt.

6. To serve, simply slice thinly with a long knife.

Note: Want to give your gravlax a subtly smoky flavor? Swap out about one-third of the kosher salt for smoked salt.

DRY-BRINED ROAST TURKEY WITH CIDER GRAVY

I know some people swear by brining. "Best turkey I've ever had!" "So moist!" "I'll never do Thanksgiving any other way!" Well, call me Debbie Downer, but I am not a fan. At least not as far as *traditional* brining goes. For one thing, making the brining solution is a holy mess. For another, the prospect of finding a vessel large enough to house that giant bird plus all the liquid it sits in is a big pain in the neck (don't even get me started on trying to find room for that vessel in my fridge during Thanksgiving week!). *But*—and there's a really big *but*—dry brining is another ball game entirely.

Dry brining involves rubbing salt, seasonings, and usually sugar directly onto a piece of meat (turkey, chicken, what-have-you) and then letting it sit in the fridge for a good, long rest before cooking.

The science behind how and why this works is kind of counterintuitive, because, as we know, salt draws out moisture through osmosis. You'd think, therefore, that salting a turkey ahead of time would make it dry, but somehow the result is just the opposite. Salt dissolves into the very juices it draws out of the meat and then becomes reabsorbed back into it, where it not only seasons the meat but also tenderizes it. Whodathunk?!

Once your turkey is brined, you can use whichever cooking method you like: deep-frying, grilling, smoking, or roasting old-school as here. You'll be inclined to rinse the bird before

Continued

cooking it—but don't! Leave it as is for the best flavor and crispiest skin. And serve it with this yummy cider-laced gravy for the ultimate fall feast.

Serves 12

TURKEY

3 tablespoons coarse sea salt

1 tablespoon freshly ground black pepper

1½ teaspoons dried herbs, such as thyme, sage, and rosemary

One 14- to-16-pound whole turkey (thawed, if previously frozen)

GRAVY

1 cup hard cider or apple cider

2 to 3 cups low-sodium chicken stock

4 tablespoons olive oil or unsalted butter

⅓ cup all-purpose flour

1. Prepare the turkey: Mix the coarse salt, pepper, and herbs together in a small bowl.

2. Pat the outside of the turkey dry with paper towels.

3. Sprinkle the salt mixture on all surfaces of the turkey, including the cavity.

4. Place the turkey, breast side up, in a rimmed baking sheet or roasting pan and refrigerate, uncovered, for 3 days.

5. To cook the turkey, remove it from the refrigerator and leave it at room temperature for at least 1 hour. Preheat the oven to 425°F.

6. Place the turkey, breast side up, on a roasting rack in a roasting pan. Roast for 30 minutes, then lower the oven temperature to 325°F and continue to roast until a thermometer inserted in the deepest part of the thigh reads 165°F, 2½ to 3 hours total.

7. Remove the turkey from the oven, transfer it to a platter or carving board, and tent it with foil. Let it rest for 30 minutes.

8. Meanwhile, make the gravy: Strain the drippings into a bowl. Let stand for 5 minutes, then skim off and discard the fat.

9. Place the empty roasting pan across two burners over medium-high heat. Add the cider and cook for 1 minute, scraping up all the browned bits stuck to the pan. Pour the cider and reserved pan drippings into a large measuring cup and add enough chicken stock to make a total of 4 cups.

10. Place the olive oil in a large saucepan and heat over medium heat (if using butter, until melted). Add the flour and cook, whisking, until golden, for 4 to 5 minutes. Whisk in the stock mixture and bring to a boil. Lower the heat and simmer until thickened, about 10 minutes.

11. Carve the turkey and serve with the gravy.

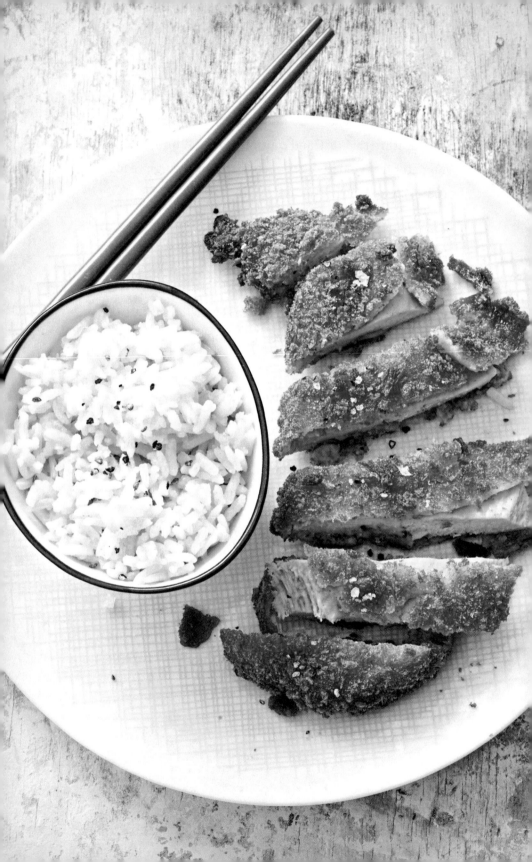

KATSU-ISH CHICKEN (A.K.A. CRISPY CHICKEN)

I have two kids who are, thankfully, both pretty open to eating all sorts of foods. One comes by it naturally—she has always loved smoked trout, olives, and mountains of beans. The other has come a long way, but if we hadn't intervened early to help her explore a variety of foods, she likely would have traces of breaded chicken product embedded in her DNA by this point. Which is to say that I know my way around a chicken cutlet. This version has always been a winner with my family and is definitely on the greatest hits album for my personal chef business—clients request my Crispy Chicken all the time. Here, it's pounded thin, dredged in flour, beaten egg, and panko (Japanese bread crumbs), and then fried. What's not to love?

The recipe is a nod to a traditional Japanese comfort classic—hence the panko—that's often served with shredded cabbage, rice, sunomono (Japanese pickles), and a sweet-salty sauce called tonkatsu sauce. It's pretty straightforward, but I use two tricks that make all the difference here: (1) salting the cutlets generously ahead of time to improve their texture and flavor (for the science behind this, see Dry-Brined Roast Turkey, page 89) and (2) frying them in olive oil—a decidedly inauthentic yet delicious element, hence the *-ish* in Katsu-ish Chicken. The recipe is easily doubled so you can prep a batch and freeze it for your future self.

Serves 4

Continued

1½ pounds chicken cutlets, about ¼ inch thick

Coarse sea salt

Freshly ground black pepper

¾ cup all-purpose flour

3 large eggs, beaten

2 cups panko

¼ cup olive oil

Flaky sea salt for serving

1. Season the cutlets generously with coarse salt and pepper and let them rest in the refrigerator, covered, for at least 1 hour and up to overnight.

2. Place the flour, eggs, and panko in separate shallow bowls; season each component with salt and pepper. Dip the chicken into the flour and then the egg, shaking off any excess. Then dip into the panko, pressing to adhere.

3. Heat the oil in a large skillet over medium heat. Add the chicken and cook until golden brown and cooked through, 4 to 6 minutes per side. Transfer to a paper towel–lined plate and season with flaky salt.

4. Slice the chicken into thin strips and serve immediately with shredded cabbage, white rice, Japanese pickles, and tonkatsu sauce. Or, you know, ketchup and fries. You do you.

Note: To make your own cutlets from boneless, skinless chicken breasts: Cut the chicken breasts in half horizontally. Working with one piece of chicken at a time, place in a large resealable plastic bag and pound with a rolling pin, the flat side of a meat mallet, or a small, heavy skillet until ¼ inch thick. That's it!

SEARED FLANK STEAK WITH CHIMICHURRI SAUCE

Flank steak, with its rich beefy flavor, tender flesh, and quick cooking time, is a no-brainer when it comes to fast and easy meal prep. There are just three things to keep in mind to make yours a slam dunk: (1) season the steak like crazy, (2) get the pan screaming hot, and (3) serve it with a killer sauce.

As for that sauce, Argentinean chimichurri is almost always my pick. Bright, bold, herbal, and addictive—thanks to a ton of parsley, garlic, and silky, fruity olive oil—it is the perfect complement to that beefy steak flavor. In Argentina, chimichurri is as common as ketchup is in America—it's most commonly served with red meat, but you'll find that it's good on pretty much anything: poultry, shellfish, sandwiches, vegetables, eggs . . . I almost always double or triple the sauce recipe, either because I'm feeding a crowd and/or just thinking ahead to a busy weeknight down the road (it freezes really well).

Serves 4

Continued

STEAK

One 1½-pound skirt steak, about ½ inch thick, cut in half crosswise

Sea salt and freshly ground black pepper

2 tablespoons vegetable oil

CHIMICHURRI

3 garlic cloves, minced

1 shallot, finely chopped

¼ cup red wine vinegar

¼ cup fresh lemon juice

2 cups packed fresh cilantro leaves

1 cup packed fresh flat-leaf parsley leaves

⅓ cup packed fresh oregano leaves

¾ cup extra virgin olive oil

½ teaspoon ground coriander

½ teaspoon ground cumin

1 teaspoon coarse sea salt

1. Salt the steak: Season the steak generously with sea salt and let sit at room temperature for 30 minutes.

2. Meanwhile, make the chimichurri: Combine the garlic, shallot, vinegar, and lemon juice in a small bowl and set aside for 10 minutes.

3. Transfer the garlic mixture to a blender or to a food processor fitted with a blade attachment. Add the fresh herbs and pulse to finely chop. With the motor running, drizzle

in the olive oil in a thin stream. Add the coriander, cumin, and coarse salt. Pulse once or twice to combine. Set aside.

4. Pat the steak dry with paper towels and season again with sea salt and pepper.

5. Heat a large cast-iron skillet or other heavy-bottomed pan over medium-high heat until hot. Add the vegetable oil and heat until it is shimmering and just on the verge of smoking. Add one of the steak halves to the pan and cook until nicely browned, 3 to 4 minutes per side for medium-rare.

6. Remove the steak from the pan and transfer it to a surface to rest for about 10 minutes. Repeat with the remaining steak half.

7. Once it's rested, slice the steak thinly against the grain into thin strips. Season with the coarse salt and pepper to taste and serve slathered with chimichurri sauce.

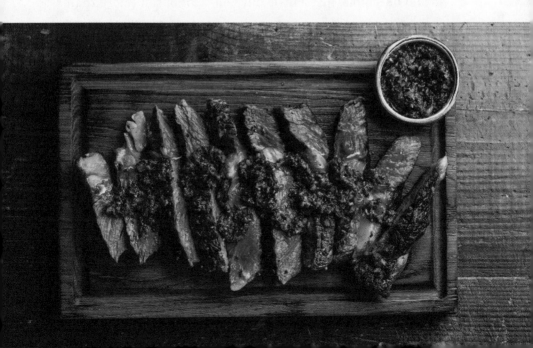

(YET ANOTHER) PERFECT ROAST CHICKEN

Roast chicken—the ultimate comfort food—is an incredibly simple undertaking and, in my opinion, something pretty much every (nonvegetarian) cook should learn how to make. And yet, I find that so often people are intimidated by it, which is probably why grocery store rotisserie chicken is now so ubiquitous. Perhaps it's because just about every chef and cookbook author has an opinion on how to make the "perfect" roast chicken. Brine it for the moistest meat. Make a spice rub—no, an herb butter. Spatchcock it for the most even cooking. Dry the skin with a hairdryer for the crispiest skin. (Seriously, I've tried that one!) From oven temperature to cooking time to basting (or not), there are a lot of chicken ideas out there!

But if you want to know the true secret to making delicious roast chicken, don't mess with it too much! Roast chicken should be simple. Just a little olive oil, a lot of salt (more than you think you should use), and some pepper is all you really *need* to roast a chicken. I happen to like bringing some lemon and garlic to the party, but if you skip that step below, you're still going to end up with a really nice chicken that's ready to become dinner, leftovers, and whatever else you've got up your sleeve. Just remember: chicken is done when it reaches 165°F on a meat thermometer in the thickest part of the thigh.

Makes 1 roast chicken

One 5- to 6-pound chicken, at room temperature,
   giblets removed

Olive oil

Sea salt

Freshly ground black pepper

1 lemon, halved

4 garlic cloves

1. Preheat the oven to 450°F.

2. Pat the chicken dry with paper towels, then rub a thin layer of olive oil all over the skin. Season the cavity and skin very generously with sea salt and pepper. Use more salt than you think you need. Stuff the cavity of the chicken with the lemon and garlic cloves.

3. Place the chicken, breast side up, in a roasting pan.

4. Lower the oven temperature to 400°F and roast the chicken, undisturbed, for an hour to an hour and a half, until it registers 165°F in the thickest part of the thigh and the juices run clear.

5. Remove from the oven and let the chicken rest for about 15 minutes, then carve and serve.

BEEF TENDERLOIN BAKED IN A SALT CRUST

I'm going to need you to trust me here, because what I'm about to say is going to sound absolutely bananas, but I promise[*] it is sound advice. One of the very best ways to cook beef tenderloin is to bake it wrapped in a completely inedible dough made of almost 50 percent salt. That's right, I want you to go out and buy one of the most expensive cuts of meat you can get your hands on, one you'd probably only serve for a special occasion, and I want you to wrap it in an inedible salt dough (a distant relative of huff paste, which is an old-timey mixture of salt, flour, and water that was used to protect meat from the heat of an open spit.) I want you to bake it in the oven until it is rock hard and then I want you to throw away that dough, because—again—it is absolutely inedible. And this procedure, I allege, is going to result in a most delicious meal.

Here's the deal: the salty dough here is almost like cement mix or mortar and—when baked—it hardens, creating something like a kiln, where moisture and flavor become locked in. And because all the meat's insanely flavorful juices simply can't leak out, that pricey tenderloin is guaranteed to be moist, perfectly medium-rare, and 100 percent holiday meal–worthy. The one thing to keep in mind is that the dough does require a little bit of advance planning—it'll need to rest for 2 to 24

---

[*] "Promises and pie-crust are made to be broken." —Jonathan Swift (1667–1745)

hours—so work that into your timetable. Otherwise, this is actually a very straightforward preparation.

Serves 8

2 cups plus 2 tablespoons coarse salt

¼ cup plus 3 tablespoons fresh thyme leaves

¼ cup plus 3 tablespoons fresh rosemary leaves

2 large eggs, separated

⅔ cup plus 2 teaspoons water

2 to 2½ cups all-purpose flour, plus more for dusting

One 2- to 3-pound beef tenderloin, tied, at room temperature

2 tablespoons extra virgin olive oil

10 fresh sage leaves

2 dried bay leaves

1 cup fresh flat-leaf parsley leaves

6 garlic cloves, thinly sliced

Freshly ground black pepper

1. Combine 2 cups of the coarse salt with 3 tablespoons of the thyme and 3 tablespoons of the rosemary in the bowl of a stand mixer fitted with the paddle attachment. Add the egg whites and water; mix until thoroughly incorporated. A little at a time, add up to 2 cups of flour, beating on medium speed, until you achieve a firm, smooth dough, for 2 to 3 minutes. Pat the dough into a square. Wrap it in plastic wrap and let it rest at room temperature at least 2 hours and up to 24 hours.

Continued

2. Preheat the oven to 375°F. Pat the tenderloin dry with paper towels. Heat the olive oil in a large skillet over medium-high heat. When the skillet is hot, add the beef. Sear on all sides, about 1½ minutes per side. Transfer to a platter or cutting board and allow to cool for 5 minutes.

3. On a lightly floured surface, roll out the dough to a rectangle that is large enough to completely encase the tenderloin. Sprinkle the remaining 2 tablespoons of coarse salt, ¼ cup of thyme, ¼ cup of rosemary and the sage, bay leaves, parsley, and garlic over the dough. Remove the twine from the tenderloin and roll the dough around beef, completely encasing it. Press the edges together to seal. Carefully transfer the wrapped beef to a roasting pan. Mix the egg yolks with 2 teaspoons of water in a small bowl; brush the entire surface of dough with egg wash.

4. Roast the dough-encased tenderloin until the crust is light golden and an instant-read thermometer inserted into the center registers 125° to 130°F, for medium-rare. Remove the pan from the oven and let the meat rest at room temperature for 1 hour. (Note: The salt crust traps in a good deal of heat and will stay warm for a very long time.)

5. When ready to serve, slice off the crust at one end and slide the beef out of the crust. Discard the crust. Season the beef with pepper, slice, and serve.

HOME-CURED CORNED BEEF

When your family finds you in the kitchen, elbow deep in salt, sugar, and mustard seeds, and asks you what you're making, they are likely to become elated when you tell them it's home-made corned beef. However, when they ask you, "When will it be ready?" and you answer, "About a week," they may feel that's a bit too long to wait for dinner. To avoid the ensuing rage and revolt, you may want to be prepared with some alternative responses, such as, "Hey, what's that over there?" and "Look, something shiny!" or—if all else fails—"Want some ice cream?" They'll soon forget all about having to wait *a whole week* for the simple-yet-delicious corned beef that you've made with your own two hands. Of course, you, too, may be wondering why it takes so freaking long to make your own, and the answer is that it's a two-part process: there's the curing and then the cooking.

First, you'll rub a brisket (the very best you can afford, please) with a blend of spices, salt, and possibly even curing salt to give it corned beef's characteristic flavor and color (more on that in the note below) and let it cure for 5 to 7 days or so. Then, you'll cook it low and slow, until it's perfectly tender, and let it cool overnight before you slice it thin and present it to your appreciative and adoring family who will be very hungry, having waited so long for this homemade delicacy. Hooray, you're a hero!

Serves 8

Continued

¾ cup coarse sea salt

1½ teaspoons pink salt (see note)

2 tablespoons packed dark brown sugar

One 3- to 5-pound brisket

2 tablespoons whole black peppercorns

2 tablespoons yellow mustard seeds

2 tablespoons whole coriander seeds

1 tablespoon allspice berries

6 whole cloves

1 tablespoon ground ginger

Hot mustard for serving

1. Whisk together coarse salt, pink salt, and brown sugar in a small bowl until combined. Rub the mixture evenly over every surface of the brisket. Combine the peppercorns, mustard seeds, coriander seeds, allspice berries, cloves, and ginger and sprinkle the mixture evenly over both sides of the brisket, pressing it gently into the meat. Wrap tightly in plastic wrap or place in a resealable plastic bag. Refrigerate for at least 7 days, massaging and flipping once a day.

2. Remove the beef from the plastic and rinse it under cool water. Pat dry with paper towels. Place the brisket in a Dutch oven or other large pot. Add enough water to cover it by 2 inches and bring to a boil. Lower the heat, cover, and simmer until very tender, 3 to 3½ hours.

3. Once cooked, transfer the beef and cooking liquid to an airtight container and refrigerate overnight (or up to 2 days).

4. Slice the beef thinly against the grain. You can reheat it gently in a skillet with some of the reserved cooking liquid or serve chilled, like deli meat. Either way, serve it with hot mustard.

Note: "Pink salt" (not to be confused with pink Himalayan salt) is a mixture of table salt and sodium nitrite that is dyed pink to distinguish it from regular salt and is commonly used in curing meat. Not only does it inhibit the growth of some bacteria, including botulism, making it a useful preservative, it is also what gives corned beef and other cured meats their traditional red color. You can omit it, if you'd like, but be aware that your corned beef will be grayish brown, rather than pink and may not last quite as long in the fridge.

CLASSIC PASTA AGLIO E OLIO

Pasta with garlic and olive oil—it sounds too simple to be good. Just three ingredients (okay, four, because: salt)—that's hardly anything at all! And yet, it's one of the very best pasta dishes there is. It is *the* pantry meal, one you can pull together in minutes with ingredients you almost certainly have on hand. This is the meal I make when I'm too tired to make anything else, when I'm cooking for myself, or when I just need comfort. Sometimes I add a bit of crushed red pepper flakes, and/or chopped flat-leaf parsley, maybe a few anchovy fillets and perhaps some freshly grated Parmesan cheese. But mostly I like to keep it to its stripped-down simplicity, because it's perfect that way.

The star of the show is the extra virgin olive oil, so you'll want to be sure to use one of the better ones on your shelf. Any robust, bold oil you like will work here. I happen to like something fruity and pungent with a peppery finish for this dish, so I might reach for an oil that's heavy on Koroneiki olives, for example. But as long as you're using a good-quality extra virgin olive oil, you'll be in fine shape.

Serves 4

1 pound spaghetti

1 cup extra virgin olive oil

6 garlic cloves, sliced thinly

1 teaspoon crushed red pepper flakes (optional)

½ cup chopped fresh parsley (optional)

3 or 4 anchovy fillets (optional)

1. Bring a pot of salted water (remember: pasta cooking water should be "salty like the sea") to a boil. Add the spaghetti and cook until it is just shy of al dente (about 1 minute less than the package directs). Reserve the pasta cooking water.

2. While the pasta is cooking, combine half of the olive oil and garlic in a large sauté pan. On medium heat, cook the garlic just until it becomes fragrant and has barely begun to turn golden, about 2 minutes. Add the red pepper flakes (if using) to the pan and let them cook for 1 minute, then add about ½ cup of the reserved pasta water.

3. Add the cooked pasta to the sauté pan. Increase the heat to high and cook for another minute in the pan, then add the parsley and anchovy fillets (if using), and the rest of the extra virgin olive oil. Continue to cook, stirring and tossing rapidly, until a creamy, emulsified sauce comes together and coats the noodles.

4. Serve right away.

FRENCH-STYLE BEEFSTEAK TOMATO TART WITH OLIVE OIL CRUST

Boy oh boy, do I get excited about tomato season! When the first few brightly hued cherry tomatoes begin to show up at the local farmers' market, I start plotting all kinds of tomato-y endeavors, using all the gorgeous varieties of tomatoes summer will bring: salads, salsas, pasta sauces . . .

The one teensy downside to my enthusiasm for the beefsteaks is my slight tendency to overbuy. I wouldn't call it a problem exactly but having too many tomatoes does present somewhat of a predicament when they don't get eaten quickly enough, because they do start to bruise and soften. This quandary is easily solved in many ways, but one of my best-loved solutions is this delicious, French-inspired tart, made with a dead-easy olive oil crust (flavorful and surprisingly light) that you don't even have to roll out (see page 170). The Dijon mustard is there to balance the sweetness of the tomatoes and the richness of the cheese. The only thing I've left out of the recipe is the requisite glass of chilled rose—optional, but highly recommended.

Makes one 10-inch tart

Continued

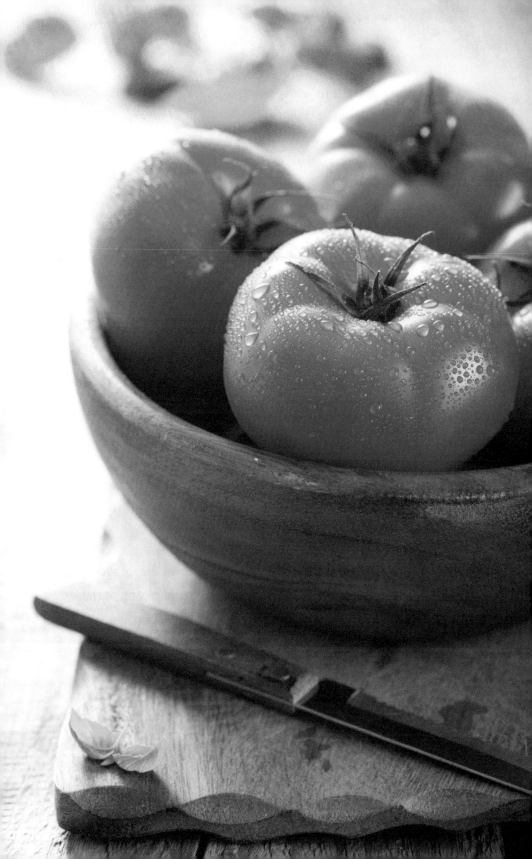

1 tablespoon Dijon or whole-grain mustard

1 unbaked olive oil tart dough (page 170; omit sugar)

6 ounces Gruyère, grated

2 to 3 large ripe tomatoes, such as beefsteak

2 tablespoons extra virgin olive oil

Sea salt and freshly ground black pepper

2 tablespoons chopped fresh herbs, such as thyme, chives, parsley, or basil

1. Preheat the oven to 425°F.

2. Spread the mustard over the bottom of the tart dough and top with half of the grated cheese, sprinkled in an even layer.

3. Slice the tomatoes and arrange them over the mustard in a single, even layer. Drizzle the olive oil over the top. Season with salt and pepper.

4. Sprinkle with half of the chopped fresh herbs, then the remaining grated cheese, and finally the rest of the fresh herbs.

5. Bake the tart for about 30 minutes, or until the tomatoes are just beginning to take on a little brown color and the crust and top layer of cheese are both golden brown.

6. Serve warm or at room temperature.

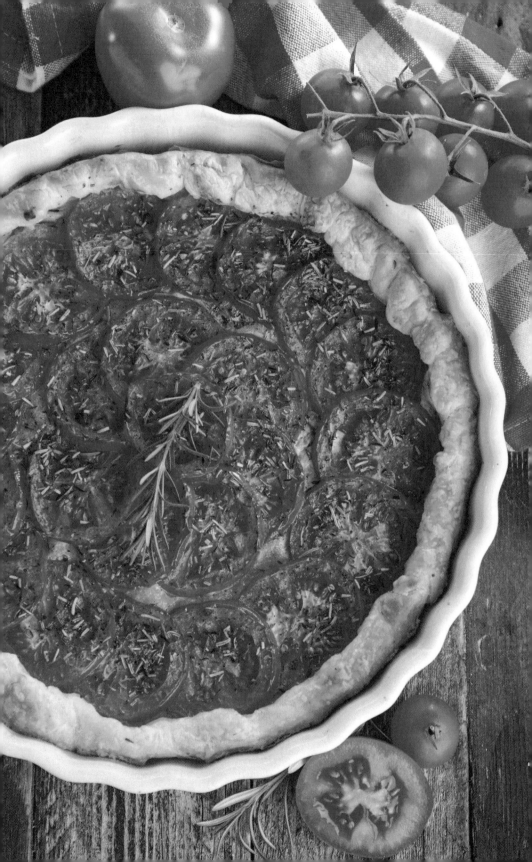

MEDITERRANEAN-STYLE BRAISED CHICKPEAS WITH OLIVES AND SUN-DRIED TOMATOES

I am a sucker for chickpeas. I could absolutely eat them every day. Mashed with lemon and garlic, roasted until crisp, pureed into a silky hummus, tossed into salads, hidden under a fried egg . . . you name it, I'm in. But my absolute favorite way to eat this pantry superstar is like this: in a steamy bath of olive oil until they're buttery soft. They're so, so good. And unbelievably easy to put together. And fun to tweak. Rather than flavoring them with a nod to the Mediterranean as I have here, add Indian spices and a dollop of yogurt or Moroccan spices and preserved lemon, or anything else that floats your boat. Whether you make this recipe as is or go your own way, you will serve these salty, spicy chickpeas with good, crusty bread or on thick slices of toast. Notice I am not gently suggesting you do so. It's a mandate. Do it! Okay, fine—the bread is optional, but don't blame me when you're sitting at the table with a beautifully flavored oil surrounding silky chickpeas and nothing to sop it all up with. You've been warned . . .

Serves 4

1 cup extra virgin olive oil

1 to 2 anchovy fillets

½ small yellow onion, minced

Two 15-ounce cans chickpeas, drained and rinsed

¼ cup thinly sliced sun-dried tomatoes

½ teaspoon coarse sea salt

Freshly ground black pepper

3 sprigs fresh oregano

½ teaspoon red pepper flakes

¼ cup cured black olives, pitted and torn

½ lemon, sliced

½ cup crumbled feta or goat cheese (optional)

Crusty bread for serving—not optional (Just kidding! Sort of.)

1. Heat the oven to 375°F.

2. Heat about 1 tablespoon of the olive oil in a large oven-proof skillet with a lid or Dutch oven over medium heat until shimmering. Add the anchovies and onion and sauté for 5 minutes, or until the anchovies dissolve and the onion is soft and just beginning to brown.

3. Add the remaining olive oil, chickpeas, sun-dried tomatoes, coarse salt, black pepper, oregano, red pepper flakes, olives, and lemon slices to the pan, then stir to combine. Cover tightly and bake for 30 to 40 minutes, until the mixture is bubbling and the chickpeas are soft.

4. Let cool slightly. Before serving, remove the oregano and season to taste as necessary with salt and pepper. Serve with crusty bread for mopping up the fragrant oil.

FANTASTIC FRIED EGG

One day when I was in culinary school, we were tasked with examining how food reacted when cooked in different fats: butter, clarified butter, brown butter, and olive oil. I remember cooking a lot of eggs, and I remember that at a certain point, we were told to fry an egg in olive oil. Now, one of the really fun aspects of going to culinary school is all of the tasting one gets to do. Typically, I would have a bite or two of a finished product or a taste of an important ingredient, get the gist, and move on to the next thing.

But, on this particular day I'd tasted the eggs cooked in butter (classic), clarified butter (delicious), and brown butter (even better), but when it came to the egg cooked in olive oil, I literally stopped in my tracks. It was that good. For one thing, it had this beautiful, crispy, lacy edge and a perfectly browned underside. But more than that, it was absolutely *full* of flavor.

Instead of merely tasting the egg, I ate the whole thing. And then I made myself another. And—*gulp*—another. Each one was rich, savory, soft, runny, and crisp all at once. A revelation. By that point, I'd been tasting eggs for the better part of two hours—a bite here, another there—and I'm not sure how many I ate that day, but, all told, it's a number that I'm sure a cardiologist would not condone.

Since then, I have happily continued to make amazing eggs fried in olive oil. They are, of course, perfect right out of the pan, but sprinkling them with a little flaky salt and freshly ground black pepper is only going to improve your day, so don't skip that step.

Makes 1 fried egg

Continued

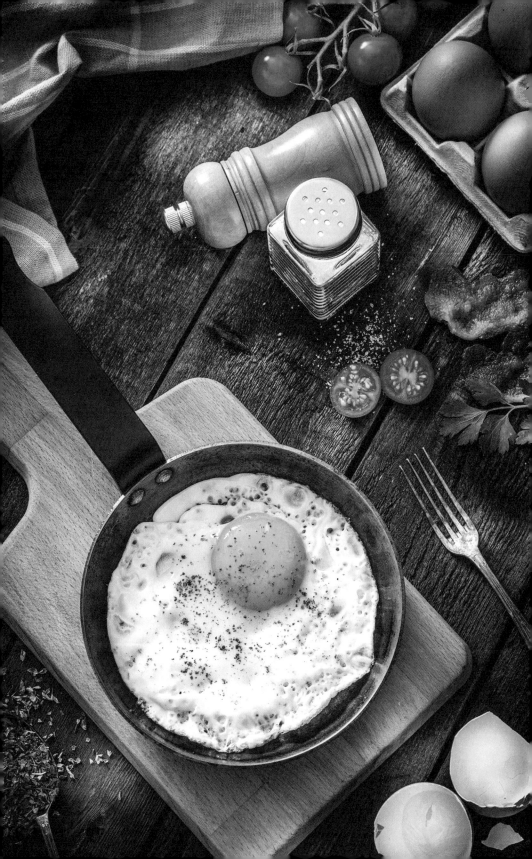

1 tablespoon extra virgin olive oil

1 large egg

Flaky sea salt

Freshly ground black pepper

1. Heat the olive oil in a small, heavy skillet over medium-high heat until it's extremely hot.

2. Crack the egg into a ramekin or small bowl. When the oil is hot, carefully pour the egg into the pan and lower the heat to medium-low. Be careful—it will almost certainly splatter.

3. Cook the egg, tilting the pan occasionally and/or basting it in oil with a spoon, until the edges are crisp and golden and the yolk is just barely set, about 2 minutes.

4. Serve sprinkled with a bit of flaky salt and freshly ground black pepper.

ULTIMATE UMAMI PIZZA

Everybody loves pizza. We all know *that*. But why? Is it the stringy, salty cheese? The chewy crust? The sweet and tangy tomato sauce? Well, yes, yes, and yes. But it may also be something a bit harder to pinpoint. *Umami*, a Japanese word meaning "savory" or "deliciousness," is the fifth basic taste (along with sweet, sour, bitter, and salty) and is stimulated by the amino acid glutamate. The more glutamate in a food, the more umami it is.

Tomatoes and aged cheese are two foods that just so happen to be packed with glutamate and they also just so happen to be the building blocks of pizza. Pizza is irresistible because it is umami. There's a sort of lingering deliciousness with umami, and even a simple plain slice—my favorite—brings it. But, say you wanted to make pizza's deliciousness linger longer? The trick would be to add more umami in the form of well-chosen toppings. Not surprisingly, some of the most classic pizza toppings, such as olives, garlic, mushrooms, Parmesan, and cured meats, are high in glutamate. That said, when constructing a delicious, umami-heavy pizza, balance is key, and dumping on *all* the umami at once isn't the way to go. Stick to two or three toppings for the best results. Here, I've pulled together a handful of umami-rich toppings, including the mind-blowing porcini salt on page 46, that work well together in terms of flavor and texture to bring you a pizza with a whole lot of *something-something*.

Makes two 10-inch pizzas

Continued

1 pound pizza dough, homemade or store-bought (see note)

1 tablespoon extra virgin olive oil, plus more for brushing

6 ounces shiitake mushrooms, sliced (about 3 cups)

Sea salt and freshly ground black pepper

1 cup pizza sauce (see note)

1½ cups smoked mozzarella, shredded or sliced thinly

½ cup grated Parmesan

8 thin slices prosciutto

Porcini Salt (page 46)

1. Preheat the oven to 500°F. Divide the dough in half and cover each half with a clean kitchen towel or piece of plastic wrap.

2. Heat the olive oil in a medium skillet over medium-high heat. Add the mushrooms and sauté, stirring occasionally, until tender, about 2 minutes. Season with ¼ teaspoon of sea salt and a pinch of pepper.

3. Brush a very thin layer of olive oil on a baking sheet. Working with one half of the dough at a time, press it into a large disk with your hands and place it on the oiled baking sheet. Use your hands or a rolling pin to flatten the dough until it is about ¼ inch thick.

4. Spoon half of the pizza sauce onto the center of the dough and use the back of a spoon to spread it out to the edges. Layer on half of the mushrooms, half of the prosciutto, and half of the cheese.

5. Place the baking sheet in the oven. Bake until the crust is golden brown and the cheese is melted and browned in spots, about 10 minutes.

6. Transfer the pizza to a cutting board, let it cool slightly, then slice and serve with a sprinkling of porcini salt.

7. Repeat with the remaining dough, sauce, cheese, and toppings.

Note: No need to make your own dough here, although you most certainly can! Store-bought is fine. In fact, if you swing by your local pizza place and ask the staff to sell you a pound or two of theirs, they usually will. You can also turn this recipe into a personal pizza party by picking up packaged naan from the grocery store or even freshly baked from your favorite Indian restaurant.

As for the sauce, feel free to use a good-quality store-bought pizza sauce in a pinch, but you can also make a quick sauce yourself in about 2 minutes flat: Toss 4 garlic cloves, one 14½-ounce can of whole or diced tomatoes, 2 tablespoons of olive oil, ½ teaspoon of sugar, ¾ teaspoon of sea salt, plus freshly ground black pepper to taste into a blender and process until pureed.

Sips and Savory Snacks

CLASSIC MARGARITA (WITH SUPER EASY VARIATIONS)

I'm rarely one to turn up my nose at a smart shortcut in the kitchen, but I definitely draw the line at way-too-sweet, bottled "margarita mix." The thing is, making margaritas from scratch is pretty darn easy (you really need only three ingredients) and the end result is so superior that it's barely even worthy of comparison. Tart, crisp, just-sweet-enough, and *strong*, there's a reason the classic margarita is so well loved.

On the rocks, with salt is how I like 'em (and if you *really* want to know what I think . . . it's the only way to drink a marg), so that's what this recipe will give you. Yes, you can blend yours with ice if you absolutely *must* (I get it—my husband is on Team Frozen), but no matter what, you shouldn't skip the salted rim. Salt, as we know, isn't just for looks. It's a flavor enhancer, and a salted rim actually plays an important role in balancing the flavors of your margarita. For one thing, it helps temper any bitterness the tequila may be giving off, and it enhances both the drink's sweet and sour notes. As for the tequila, either *blanco* (a.k.a. silver) or *reposado* will work. Blanco is less aged tequila and will give you a crisper cocktail, but if you want a bit more complexity, go for reposado, which is darker in color and has been aged in oak.

Serves 2

Coarse sea salt for rimming glasses

Lime wedges for rims and garnish

4 ounces tequila (blanco or reposado)

2 ounces orange liqueur, such as Cointreau or triple sec

2 ounces fresh lime juice

Ice

1. Fill a small dish with a few tablespoons of coarse salt. Run a lime wedge around the outer rims of two rocks glasses and dip the rims in the salt. Set aside.

2. Combine the tequila, Cointreau, and lime juice in a cocktail shaker. Fill the shaker the rest of the way with ice and shake until the outside of the shaker is frosty, about 15 seconds.

3. Fill the glasses with fresh ice, being careful not to disturb the salted rims, and strain margarita into both glasses. Garnish with lime wedges and serve.

Continued

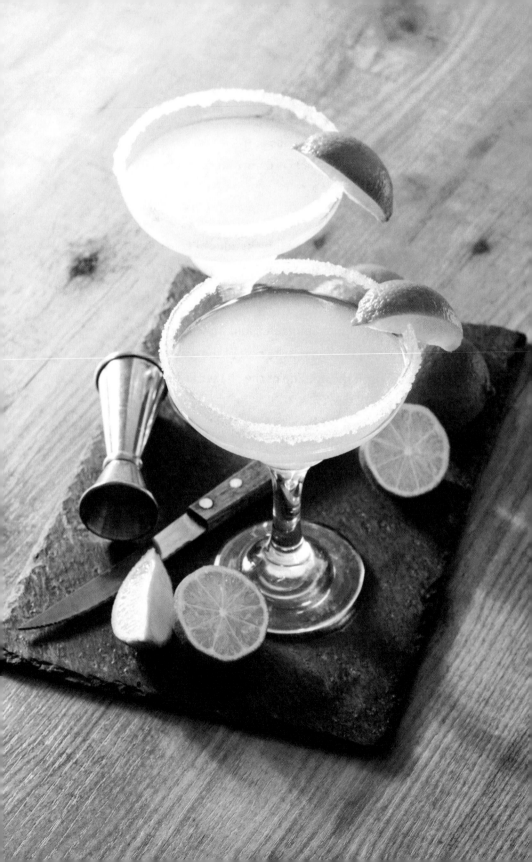

HOW TO TAKE YOUR CLASSIC MARGARITA TO THE NEXT LEVEL

Add fresh fruit. You can use pretty much any other citrus juice in place of the lime for a twist on the classic margarita. (Twist. Get it?) Grapefruit is especially delicious, as are tangerine, blood orange, and Meyer lemon. Lots of other fruit works well, too, and can be added in conjunction with lime—mango, strawberry, and watermelon play well here. Adding a bit of pureed grilled fruit, such as peaches and pineapple, brings out the smokiness of aged tequila for a sophisticated spin.

. . . or vegetables! Really! Cucumber—juiced, grated, or even just popped in as a garnish—adds a refreshing twist to the drink. And, believe it or not, beet juice has been known to show up in margaritas from time to time. Earthy and sweet, the flavor of beets actually works quite well against the sharp, sour background of lime and tequila. Creamy, cool avocado is a welcome addition, too, lending a smooth, silky texture to a frozen margarita.

Garnish with flavored salts. Many of the flavored salts in chapter 1 of this book would work beautifully on the rim of a margarita glass, bringing another layer of flavor to the party. Combining salt and something sweet, such as coarse sugar or sweetened, shredded coconut on the rim of the glass, can also offer a nice counterpoint to the sour flavor of margaritas. Others to try: cinnamon/sugar/salt, fresh lime zest + salt, or—one of my favorites—2 parts cocoa powder to 1 part chili powder to 1 part salt. That, on the rim of a pineapple margarita—ooh, baby!

Consider bringing some heat. From chile-infused tequila to sliced fresh jalapeño, adding a bit of something spicy to your margarita is a fun way to add flavor and interest to the drink. Add freshly ground black pepper or cayenne to the salt on your glass rim, freeze thin slices of serrano or habanero pepper in ice cubes, and add those to your rocks glass for a slow burn, or sweeten your drink with agave or simple syrup that's been steeped with hot peppers.

Add an herbal element. Fresh herbs, such as mint, cilantro, basil, rosemary, or even lavender, can bring brightness, earthiness, or floral notes that completely transform a margarita. As in . . . pear-lavender margaritas with vanilla salt (page 43) and a splash of Champagne. Black! Tie! Worthy! Or how about grapefruit-rosemary margaritas with smoked salt? That'd be great at a holiday party, no? Whether you muddle fresh herbs in the bottom of the cocktail shaker before adding the rest of the cocktail ingredients or use them to infuse a simple syrup, they're fun to play around with and delicious to sip!

CUCUMBER, SEA SALT, AND VODKA COCKTAIL

Ever notice how the water they serve at fancy spas always tastes so much better than "regular" water? With cucumber, mint, and sometimes lemon (and—if you're *really* lucky—maybe even a hibiscus bloom or jasmine blossom), it's just about the most refreshing drink ever.

As I am wont to do, I have taken things a bit too far and present you with this spa water–inspired cocktail. Refreshing and slightly savory, it tastes like the love child of an aromatherapy massage and happy hour. If you can get fresh, firm Kirby cucumbers, they're best here—sweeter and more flavorful than others—but really, any cucumber will make a delicious cocktail. And while I recommend pink salt, it's largely for the sake of the visual contrast between the blushing salt and that vibrant green cucumber. Use whichever fine salt you like. This recipe is easily scaled to make a whole pitcher; simply quadruple the ingredient quantities, muddle the cukes, ginger, and mint in a large container, then strain into a pitcher and proceed with the recipe. I mean, you've gotta stay hydrated, you know?

Serves 2

½ cup peeled and finely chopped Kirby cucumber

2 tablespoons grated fresh ginger

4 sprigs mint

Pinch of pink sea salt

1 tablespoon simple syrup (equal parts sugar and water, heated until sugar dissolves)

1 tablespoon fresh lime juice

4 ounces vodka

Ice

8 ounces sparkling water

GARNISHES

2 slices Kirby cucumber, unpeeled

Pink or other fine sea salt

A few fresh mint leaves

1. Muddle the cucumber, ginger, mint, and pink salt in the bottom of a cocktail shaker. Add the simple syrup, lime juice, and vodka. Fill the shaker with ice. Shake hard for 60 seconds.

2. Fill a highball glass halfway with ice cubes. Strain the cocktail mixture into the two glasses. Top with sparkling water.

3. Garnish each glass with a slice of unpeeled cucumber, a sprinkling of pink sea salt, and a few mint leaves. Serve.

Note: This drink is even better with mint syrup. To make, simply add a few sprigs of fresh mint to still-warm simple syrup and allow it to steep for 30 minutes!

MICHELADA

I don't think beer cocktails get the props they deserve. They're versatile, refreshing, and so very easy-drinking. Mixing beer with juice, spices, liqueurs, and other flavorings to create a downright fun libation is popular all over the world—from English shandies to German *Radlers* to Spanish *clara con limon*. A michelada is one of the most refreshing and flavorful of them all. It's almost always made with some combination of beer, fresh lime juice, and hot sauce or chili powder—boldly sour and assertively spicy, but perfectly balanced—and served with a salted rim.

There are, of course, about as many variations on a michelada recipe as there are michelada drinkers, which is to say that there's lots of room to play and customize it to your own personal taste. This recipe is inspired by my first run-in with a michelada, which I bought from a street vendor in Cuernavaca, Mexico. It's pretty no frills, but decidedly tart and spicy, which is how I like it. You can play with the ratios to suit your taste, but following a couple of simple ground rules will ensure a perfect base: (1) use a light beer, ideally a Mexican lager (such as Modelo, Pacífico, Tecate, Victoria, or Corona), and (2) fresh lime juice only!

Makes 1 drink

1 tablespoon coarse sea salt

Lime wedges

2 ounces fresh lime juice

2 teaspoons hot sauce

Ice

12 ounces light Mexican beer (see headnote)

1. Pour the coarse salt into a small, shallow dish and spread into an even layer. Wet the rim of a pint or pilsner glass with a lime wedge and dip the rim into the salt to coat.

2. Combine the lime juice and hot sauce in the bottom of the glass. Add a pinch or two of salt, fill the glass with ice, and top with beer. Stir gently and garnish with a lime wedge. Serve with the remaining beer, topping off your drink as you go.

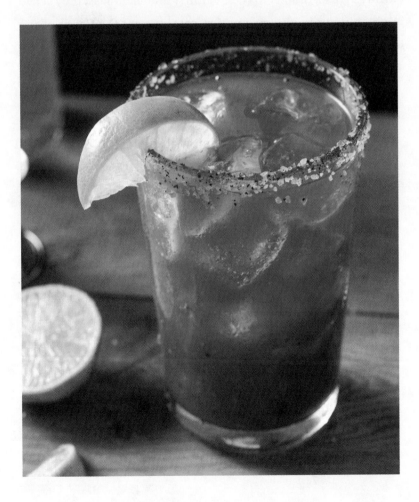

REALLY DIRTY MARTINI (AND A RECIPE FOR OIL-WASHED VODKA OR GIN)

A dirty martini is one in which a bit of brine from the olives is added to the drink to kick up that salty balance even more. Olives have long been associated with the classic martini. An ideal garnish, thanks to their salinity and brininess, they serve to highlight the gin's aromatics, complement the flavor of the vermouth, and generally balance out the drink's intensity. Because I tend to skew savory in my cocktailing, I do love a dirty martini (with apologies to mixology purists).

But what's really lovely is introducing olive oil to the mix via a process called fat-washing. I know, it sounds more like something you might do in the laundry room, but it's actually a technique that adds amazing savory flavor and a rich and velvety texture to drinks. It involves adding liquid fat (olive oil, in our case) to some kind of alcohol (here, it's vodka or gin), letting it sit for a few hours, then chilling it in the freezer until the fat solidifies and can easily be skimmed off. What's left is a spirit with a smoother texture and a silky mouthfeel rather than a strong flavor—the process tones down some of the harsher flavors and highlights the olive oil's richness and complexity. As is always the case when using just a handful of ingredients, quality is important—you're going to want to make sure you go top-notch all the way around, so reach for your best-quality booze and olive oil. And that jar of blue cheese–stuffed olives you once got in a gift basket and then shoved in the pantry? This is their day in the sun. Cheers!

Serves 2

4 ounces oil-washed vodka or gin (recipe follows)
1 ounce dry vermouth
1½ ounces olive brine
Cocktail olives for garnish

Combine the vodka or gin, vermouth, and olive brine in a mixing glass with ice. Stir to chill and strain into a chilled martini glass. Garnish with olives on a pick.

Oil-Washed Vodka or Gin

Makes about 1 cup vodka or gin

1 cup vodka or gin
¼ cup extra virgin olive oil

1. Combine the gin and olive oil in a freezer-safe container with a lid.

2. Shake vigorously and store in a cool, dark place for 24 hours.

3. Place the container in the freezer and freeze until the olive oil completely separates and solidifies.

4. Remove the olive oil layer, then strain remaining alcohol through a coffee filter to clarify.

SALTY DOG

A Salty Dog is a refreshing and simple cocktail made from grapefruit juice and vodka, served in a glass with a salted rim. Fans of *The Larry Sanders Show* will remember it as Artie's libation of choice. It is also one of about three recipes I remember learning in a bartending course I took after graduating from college.

As it turns out, I never ended up landing a bartending job, but I sure was ready to show the world my best Pink Squirrels, Rusty Nails, Golden Cadillacs, and Brandy Alexanders. Alas, the Salty Dog is one of the few from that rigorous training that I actually remember how to make—and that's a good thing, for it is pretty much sunshine in a glass, perfect for sipping on a steamy day or reminding you of summer in the dead of winter. Totally worth the investment in that postgrad education, I'd say.

Serves 2

Coarse sea salt
Ice cubes
½ cup vodka or gin
1 cup fresh grapefruit juice

1. Fill a small dish with a few tablespoons of coarse salt. Moisten the rims of two highball glasses. Gently dip rims into the salt to coat lightly.

2. Fill the glasses with ice cubes. Pour ¼ cup of vodka into each glass. Pour 1 cup of grapefruit juice into each glass. Serve.

AGUA MINERAL PREPARADA

Salt and lime—one of the most irresistible culinary combinations there is—can make even the most basic foods pop with flavor. Even sparkling water. In Mexico, where salt and lime are added to everything under the sun, you can find this combination pretty much anywhere: at restaurants, bars, even in convenience stores, where they sell a popular bottled version (Peñafiel Twist). Just a shot of lime juice, a pinch of salt, and sparkling water in a glass with a salted rim—so simple, yet so perfect. It's the ideal nonsugary, sort of fancy, almost-cocktail. It's perfect for cooling off on a hot day, for recovering after a long night of excess, or for rehydrating after a workout. As a good friend (who used to live in Mexico and who introduced me to this magical drink) so aptly put it: "There's really never a time when this isn't an appropriate drink." So true.

Makes 1 drink

⅛ teaspoon coarse sea salt, plus more for rimming the glass
Juice of ½ lime
Sparkling water

1. Pour a tablespoon or two of coarse salt into a small, shallow dish and spread into an even layer. Wet the rim of a tall glass with a lime wedge and dip the rim into the salt to coat.

2. Fill the glass with ice. Add the lime juice and ⅛ teaspoon of salt. Top with sparkling water. Serve.

BAKED OLIVE OIL AND SEA SALT TORTILLA CHIPS

I have to confess that I started making my own tortilla chips out of desperation, once upon a time when I just *had* to have chips and salsa, but didn't have any tortilla chips in the house. I did have a jar of salsa and briefly considered settling for dippers in the form of cut-up vegetables, of all things (*quelle horreur*!), but then remembered a package of corn tortillas I had in the fridge. Thank goodness! I cut them into wedges, brushed them with oil, sprinkled them with salt, and baked them until they were browned and crisp. And you know what? Not only were they delicious, but I actually liked them *better* than the chips in the bag that I didn't have. These chips tasted more like corn, for one thing, and they were a lovely combination of crisp and ever-so-slightly chewy. The one trick I learned the hard way in subsequent homemade chip endeavors is to coat the tortillas with oil *before* cutting them. Trust me, it's a lot of tedious brushing otherwise if you're making more than just one or two tortillas' worth, as I did my first time around. And go for a flaky salt here—not only will it adhere better to the chips, but it's a softer saltiness that allows both the flavors of the corn and the olive oil to shine through.

Serves 4

Twelve 6- to 8-inch corn tortillas, cut into quarters

1 tablespoon olive oil

Flaky sea salt

1. Preheat the oven to 350°F. Line two baking sheets with parchment paper.

2. Brush both sides of the tortillas with the olive oil. Stack the tortillas and cut the pile into sixths or eighths to make chips.

3. Spread the chips out in a single layer on the prepared baking sheets and season with flaky salt.

4. Bake until golden brown and crisp, about 15 minutes.

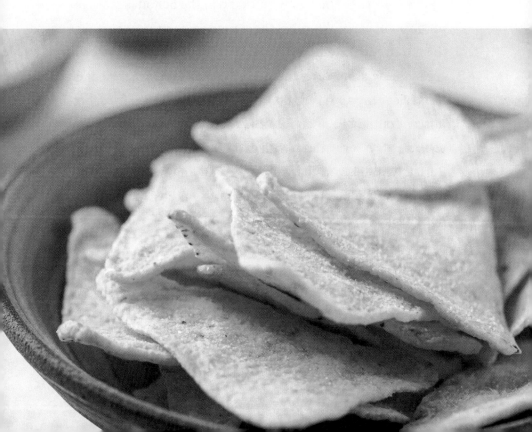

BOARDWALK FRIES

French fries, chips, steak fries, frites, curly fries, waffle fries . . .
Call them what you will, if they're crisp and golden on the outside, soft and fluffy on the inside and really well salted, I'm in. *Ask
me. PLEASE, ASK ME!* "Would you like fries with that?" *Yes! Yes I
would like fries with that!* In the hierarchy of fries, there's one that
tops the list for me: Atlantic beach–style boardwalk fries (a.k.a.
'80s shopping mall food court fries). And believe it or not, boardwalk fries—thick, hand-cut fries, served with vinegar and, often,
Old Bay seasoning—are quite possible to replicate at home.

There are a few tricks that make them work. The first is to
soak the potatoes in salted water after cutting them to remove
some of the starch and to season the fries. The second is to
double fry them. Their first quick dip in the hot oil is more for
purposes of parcooking, but the second go-round is what takes
them to french fried nirvana—evenly cooked, golden brown,
crispy perfection. Sure, there is a time and a place for baked
fries (I love my air fryer. I do.), but if you want french fries rem-
iniscent of the beach boardwalk, there is no way around it—
you gotta fry. Serve these with extra Old Bay and malt vinegar.
Purists will tell you that ketchup is a no-no with boardwalk
fries (there's almost a religion about it on East Coast beach
boardwalks), but go ahead if you like. I promise I won't tell.

Serves 4 to 6

6 cups hot water (110 to 120°F)

2 tablespoons fine sea salt, plus more for serving

6 large russet potatoes, scrubbed and peeled

Vegetable or peanut oil for deep-frying

Apple cider vinegar or malt vinegar (optional)

Old Bay seasoning (optional)

1. Combine the hot water and fine salt in a large bowl. Stir to dissolve the salt. Set aside.

2. Using a sharp knife, cut the peeled potatoes lengthwise into slabs that are about ½ inch thick. Stack the slabs and cut them into ½-inch-wide sticks. Place the cut potatoes in the bowl of salt water and soak for 15 to 30 minutes.

3. Remove the potatoes from the water, lay them out on paper towels or clean kitchen towels, and dry completely, patting off as much water as possible.

4. Heat 2 inches of oil in a heavy stockpot or Dutch oven over medium heat to 300°F on a deep-fry thermometer. Working in batches, lower the potatoes into the oil and stir to separate, using a spider or slotted spoon. Cook just until softened, about 3 minutes. Use the spider or slotted spoon to transfer the potatoes to a paper towel–lined baking sheet to drain. Repeat with the remaining potatoes.

5. Heat the oil to 350°F, and—again—working in batches, add the parcooked potatoes to the oil. Stir to separate. Cook until golden brown, 4 to 5 minutes. Transfer the fries to a paper towel–lined baking sheet to drain. Season with sea salt and vinegar, if you like, or Old Bay seasoning. Serve immediately.

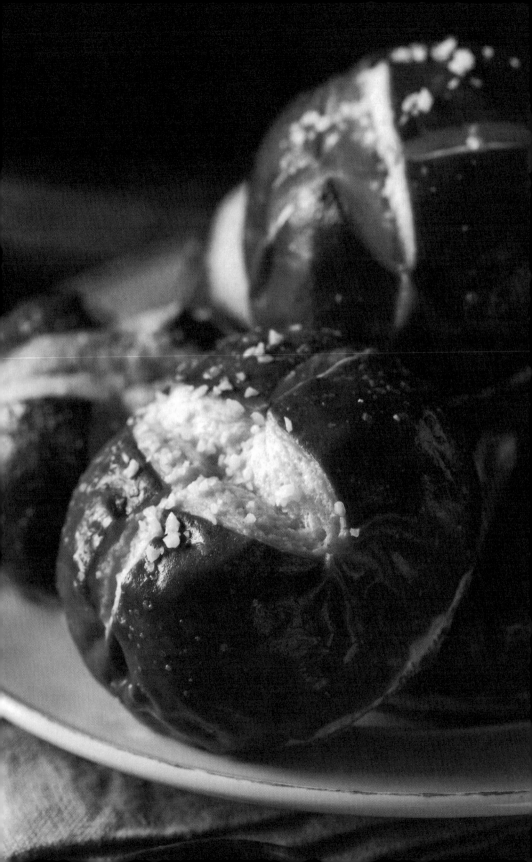

PRETZEL ROLLS

Making soft pretzels at home is much easier than you might think—even more so if you take my advice and shortcut your way through it using store-bought pizza dough (see Soft Pretzels in my book *The Baking Soda Companion*). They're a crowd-pleaser and a real treat. This recipe is even easier than making traditional soft pretzels (which are already easy!) in that it completely skips the twisting/shaping step in favor of rolling the dough into little balls. The end result is perfectly soft, chewy, salty, and pretzel-y, but shaped for a variety of serving options.

Stuff them with all manner of sandwich innards. Tear them apart and dip them into beer cheese or good mustard. Or serve them with a big bowl of soup, and you've won at dinner. I've given you the scoop on making from-scratch dough here, but you can definitely swap in a pound of store-bought pizza dough in a pinch. Truth be told, the results won't be quite as good, but no one's going to complain about them either. Know what I'm saying?

Makes 12 rolls

Continued

2¼ teaspoons instant yeast (1 packet)

1½ cups lukewarm water

¼ cup unsalted butter, melted

1 teaspoon coarse sea salt, plus more for sprinkling

1 tablespoon brown sugar

3¾ cups all-purpose flour, plus more for dusting

Butter or oil, for bowl

BAKING SODA BATH

8 cups water

½ cup baking soda

1. Combine the yeast, warm water, 2 tablespoons of the melted butter, coarse salt, brown sugar, and 3 cups of the flour in the bowl of a stand mixer fitted with the dough hook or in a large bowl. Mix the ingredients (use a wooden spoon if mixing by hand) until a shaggy dough forms. Add the remaining ¾ cup of flour and mix until the dough is no longer sticky.

2. Use the stand mixer's dough hook to knead until the dough is smooth and elastic, or turn out the dough onto a floured surface and knead by hand for 3 minutes. Shape the dough into a ball, place it in a large greased bowl, and cover tightly with plastic wrap, Allow the dough to rise in a warm place until nearly doubled in size, about an hour.

3. Once risen, punch down the dough, turn it out onto a lightly floured surface and, with a sharp knife, divide it into 12 equal pieces. Form each piece of dough into a ball.

4. Preheat the oven to 400°F. Line two baking sheets with parchment paper.

5. Prepare the baking soda bath: In a wide saucepan or Dutch oven, bring the 8 cups of water to a boil and add the baking soda. Working with two pretzel rolls at a time, boil for 30 seconds, then flip the pretzel rolls over and boil for another 30 seconds. Remove them from the water, using a slotted spoon, and place on the prepared baking sheet. Repeat with the remaining dough.

6. Lightly brush each roll with the remaining melted butter and sprinkle with coarse sea salt.

7. Bake for 22 to 26 minutes, or until deeply golden brown.

8. Remove from the oven and serve warm or cool completely on a wire rack. Store in an airtight container for up to 3 days.

DIY SALTINE CRACKERS

Saltines are surprisingly easy to make at home with nothing more than a very simple dough, a rolling pin, and a baking sheet. A pantry staple that you can make yourself—pretty cool! And just think of all the lunches, snacks, and dinners you'll be ready to embellish. Crackers and soup. Cheese and crackers. Crackers and peanut butter. This recipe is pretty fool-proof and easily customized. Although I like them best with just a sprinkling of flaky salt, it wouldn't be crazy to consider a sprinkling of seeds, herbs, or some combination of the two.

Makes about 12 dozen crackers

1 cup lukewarm water

1 tablespoon instant yeast

1 teaspoon sugar

2 tablespoons unsalted butter, at room temperature

⅓ cup olive oil, plus more for oiling bowl and greasing baking sheets

3 cups all-purpose flour

1 teaspoon kosher salt

½ teaspoon baking soda

Maldon sea salt, for sprinkling

1. Combine the water, yeast, sugar, butter, olive oil, flour, kosher salt, and baking soda using the dough hook of a stand mixer, or by hand with a wooden spoon, to form a shaggy dough. Knead (by hand or in the machine) until the dough becomes smooth and elastic, 10 to 15 minutes.

2. Lightly oil a large bowl. Form the dough into a ball and place it in the bowl, turning to coat it with oil. Cover the bowl with a clean kitchen towel or plastic wrap and let it rise until doubled in size, about 1 hour.

3. Preheat oven to 300°F. Lightly grease several baking sheets with the olive oil or line them with parchment paper.

4. Use a rolling pin to roll the dough into a large rectangle about 1/16 inch thick. Prick the dough all over with a fork. Cut into squares, circles, or whatever shape you'd like. (A pizza cutter and ruler makes this part a breeze.)

5. Transfer the crackers to the baking sheets, leaving a small space between each piece of dough.

6. Sprinkle Maldon salt on top, pressing gently with your fingers to help it adhere.

7. Bake, rotating the pans at about the 3-minute point, until just set and dry to the touch, about 5 minutes total. Lower the oven temperature to 250°F. Bake, rotating the pans at about the 12-minute point, until golden brown and crisp, 25 to 35 minutes.

8. Remove from the oven and let cool completely on the baking sheets set on wire racks.

9. Store in an airtight container for several weeks.

MARINATED FETA IN OLIVE OIL

Feta, it turns out, is a bit like Champagne or scotch. You can't call it feta if it isn't from Greece. If you are a scotch drinker, feta is to white brined cheese what scotch is to whiskey. So, there's your fun feta fact. Thankfully, though, this impressive and incredibly simple appetizer/snack works fine with just about any salty cheese—I don't care what you call it! So, feel free to skip the feta and go for queso fresco, halloumi, or fresh mozzarella. Even chèvre would be delicious, although you wouldn't get quite the same saltiness that you'll have with one of the others listed. However you choose to go, what you'll end up with is salty chunks of cheese infused with fruity olive oil and fresh herbs.

This is a great snack served on crackers or toast with an adult beverage (sparkling wine, perhaps?), or simply as a topping to jazz up a salad. This is an instance when you don't need to use your very best, most expensive olive oil. You'll be adding so much flavor to the olive oil—more so every day—that you can get away with using something a bit less than top-of the-line. And when you come to the end of the cheese, you can use that leftover olive oil from the jar to make a *killer* vinaigrette.

Serves 6 to 8

8 ounces feta cheese, drained, patted dry, and cut into ½-inch cubes

2 sprigs fresh thyme or rosemary

2 wide strips lemon zest, removed with a vegetable peeler

1 bay leaf

1 teaspoon whole black peppercorns

½ teaspoon red pepper flakes (optional)

1 cup extra virgin olive oil

1. Put the cheese into a pint glass jar.

2. Tuck the fresh herbs, lemon zest, bay leaf, peppercorns, and red pepper flakes (if using) into the jar, and then cover the contents with the oil.

3. Seal tightly and chill for at least 2 days or up to 1 week.

4. Bring to room temperature before serving.

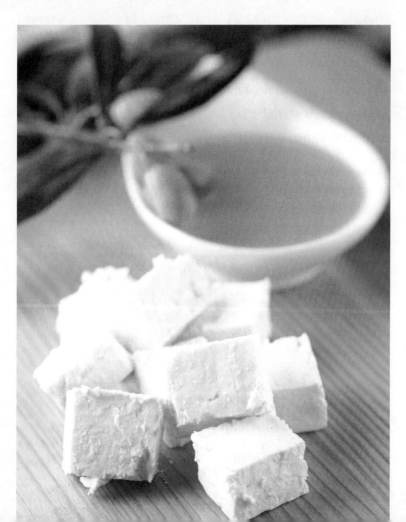

HOMEMADE SALTED BUTTER

Believe it or not, to make your very own butter at home, all you need is a stand mixer, a pint of cream, and a pinch of salt and not—as you may have assumed—a butter churn, a cow, and a Laura Ingalls Wilder–style bonnet. (Although you should feel free to wear what*ever* gets you in the mood to cook!) Over the course of about 15 minutes, you'll watch cream become whipped cream become butter. Right before your eyes, like actual magic! It's a great project to do with kids—even better if you skip the stand mixer and let them go to town shaking (and shaking and shaking) up the cream in a mason jar until it separates. It's pretty thrilling to behold, no matter which method you use. Be sure to use good-quality cream for your butter and, if possible, avoid "ultrapasteurized" cream, which has been pasteurized at such high temperatures that the flavor is largely zapped.

Makes about 1 cup butter

1 pint heavy cream
¾ teaspoon fine sea salt

1. Combine the cream and ½ teaspoon of the fine salt in the bowl of a stand mixer fitted with the paddle attachment, or in a food processor. If using a stand mixer, cover the top with plastic wrap or a kitchen towel to prevent splattering.

2. Beat at medium-high speed, keeping an eye on its progress. After about 2 minutes, you will see that the cream has begun to resemble whipped cream. In about 3 minutes, it'll start to become stiff. Keep whipping for 2 to 3 minutes more, until you achieve a solid mass (butter) separated from liquid (buttermilk). Keep that plastic wrap or towel securely in place, because you will likely have some serious splattering at this point.

3. Pour off the buttermilk and scrape the butter into a bowl of very cold water—about ½ cup of ice water should do the trick. Sprinkle the remaining ¼ teaspoon of sea salt over the butter. Using your hands or a spatula, squeeze and knead the butter to release the buttermilk. The ice water will quickly become cloudy. Pour off the cloudy water, add another ½ cup of ice water to the bowl, and repeat the kneading/squeezing/rinsing process until the water is clear, likely after five to seven changes of water.

4. Remove the butter from the ice water and pat it dry, using paper towels or a clean dish towel. Pack the butter into an airtight container, or roll it into a log or shape it into a stick, using wax paper or parchment paper. Refrigerate for about 3 weeks or freeze for up to 3 months.

Sweets

SEA-SALTED CHOCOLATE TRUFFLES

These truffles—bite-sized chocolate confections made from ganache (a mixture of melted chocolate and warmed cream), rolled, and coated with chocolate and a sprinkle of flaky sea salt—are pretty mind-blowing and very easy to make. A sprinkling of light, crunchy sea salt. That's right. Seems unlikely, yes—but it's everything!

The salt subtly enhances the chocolate, tempers its sweetness, and balances its bitterness. Its crispy crunch against the velvety smooth interior of the truffle adds textural interest, too. It's an intense and delightful little package. Straight-up flaky salt is delicious atop these truffles and you needn't use anything else, but it's worth mentioning that this could be the perfect time to play with some of those flavored salts you've made. Vanilla salt (page 43), lavender salt (page 44), and any sort of orange or other citrus salt (page 50) would be lovely, but if you're feeling funky, give smoked salt a try or even sriracha salt (page 47) for a real "wow" effect.

Makes 12 truffles

12 ounces dark chocolate (something in the 60–70% cacao
   range), chopped
½ cup heavy cream
Flaky sea salt

1. Put 8 ounces of the chopped chocolate in a medium bowl.

2. Microwave the cream in a small microwave-safe bowl on
   HIGH for 30 to 45 seconds or in a small saucepan over low
   heat until hot but not boiling.

3. Pour the hot cream over the chopped chocolate and let
   it stand for 5 minutes, then whisk the cream and chocolate together until smooth. Refrigerate until firm, 30 to
   45 minutes.

4. Using a tablespoon or small cookie scoop, divide the
   ganache into twelve 1-ounce portions. Run your hands
   under cold water, pat dry, and then roll each portion of
   ganache into a smooth ball. Place the balls on a plate or
   baking sheet. Refrigerate for a few minutes to firm up.

5. Meanwhile, microwave the remaining 4 ounces chopped
   chocolate or heat it in a small saucepan over low heat until
   it is melted, thick, and shiny. Use a chocolate-dipping tool
   or two forks to dip the truffles in the melted chocolate,
   setting them on a piece of parchment paper.

6. Immediately, as you make them, sprinkle just the top of
   each truffle with a bit of flaky salt. Store at room temperature for up to 1 day or refrigerated for up to 2 weeks.

BREAD WITH CHOCOLATE, OLIVE OIL, AND SALT

Okay, people—listen: this toasted bread, smeared with dark chocolate, drizzled with olive oil and sprinkled with flaky salt needs to become part of your life, if it hasn't already. Inspired by something similar served at tapas bars all over Spain, it is the ideal combination of sweet, salty, bitter (in a good way), crunchy, and velvety smooth. Whether served as a decadent snack, as dessert (with a scoop of vanilla ice cream, of course), or—dare I suggest it—as, perhaps, the perfect accompaniment to your first cup of morning coffee, these utterly simple, rich, and delicious little toasts are where it's at.

Use the very best-quality ingredients you can—there are so few here, you'll taste every little nuance. When choosing your olive oil, go with something a bit more robust, as anything too subdued will be overpowered by the chocolate.

Serves 4

4 large slices crusty bread, ideally something rustic or
    country-style

6 ounces dark chocolate (at least 70% cacao), roughly chopped

2 teaspoons extra virgin olive oil

½ teaspoon flaky or coarse sea salt

1. Preheat the oven to 325°F. Arrange the slices of bread on a dry baking sheet and toast until they're golden brown on both sides, about 8 minutes.

2. Divide the chocolate evenly among the pieces of bread, leaving a ½-inch margin around the edges. Return the bread slices to the oven for 1 to 2 minutes, or until the chocolate starts to melt.

3. Remove from the oven, drizzle with the oil, and sprinkle with the flaky salt. Serve.

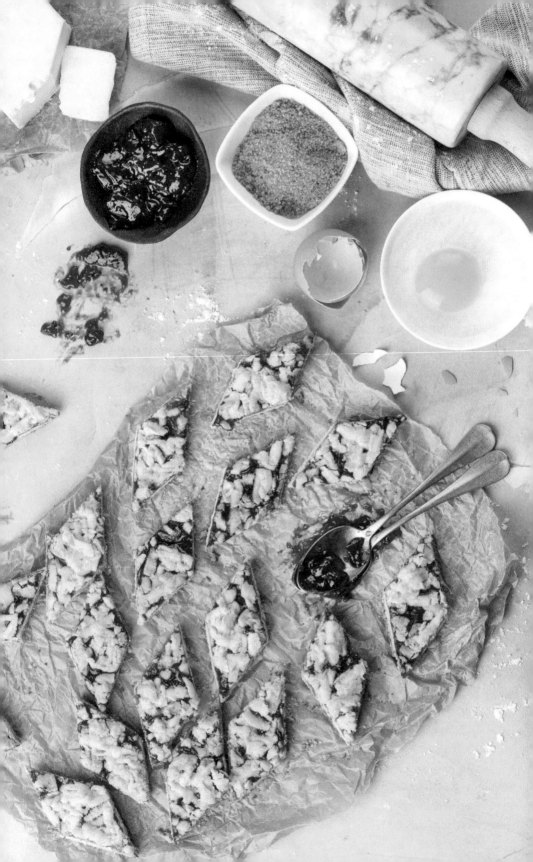

PEANUT BUTTER AND JELLY BARS

This recipe takes the classic sweet-and-salty lunchbox combination and turns it into an irresistibly sweet treat. These bars make a great after-school snack and travel well, deeming them a handy dessert to take along to potlucks and picnics. I happen to like raspberry jam best in my PB&J, but you can use whatever brings you back—strawberry, grape, apricot . . . go for what you like. And speaking of substitutions, just about any nut or seed butter works here, so if you're peanut-free, you can use almond or cashew butter and chopped almonds or cashews; or if you are tree nut–free, sunflower seed or soy nut butter.

A word of warning: it is *very* hard to wait for these little nuggets of love to cool before diving in. The thing is, they are much easier to cut neatly when they've cooled, so if you care what they look like on a serving platter, dig deep inside yourself and find the resolve to wait it out. But if looks don't matter and you want to eat them warm, that is a strong choice, too. Either way, you won't be sorry.

Makes about 36 bars

Continued

½ pound (2 sticks) unsalted butter, at room temperature, plus more for pan

1½ cups sugar

2 large eggs

1 teaspoon pure vanilla extract

2½ cups smooth peanut butter (see previous page for substitutions)

3 cups all-purpose flour

1 teaspoons coarse sea salt

1 teaspoon baking powder

1½ cups raspberry jam

⅔ cup salted peanuts, roughly chopped (see headnote)

½ teaspoon flaky sea salt

1. Preheat the oven to 350°F. Butter a 9-by-13-inch baking pan and line the bottom with parchment paper.

2. Place the butter and sugar in the bowl of a stand mixer fitted with the paddle attachment, or use a large bowl and an electric hand mixer. Cream until fluffy, about 2 minutes. With the machine running, add the eggs, one at a time. Add the peanut butter and vanilla and beat until incorporated, about 2 minutes.

3. Whisk together the coarse salt, baking powder, and flour in a small bowl. With the mixer on low speed, slowly add the flour mixture to the peanut butter mixture just until incorporated. Transfer two-thirds of peanut butter dough

to the prepared pan; spread evenly, using a spatula or your hands, then spread evenly with the jam. Drop dollops of the remaining peanut butter dough on top of jam. Sprinkle with the peanuts and flaky salt.

4. Bake until golden, about 45 minutes. Transfer to a wire rack to cool in the pan; cut into about thirty-six 1½-by-2-inch pieces.

POTATO CHIP COOKIES

You may or may not know this, but putting potato chips in cookies is a thing. And, yes, I know that putting potato chips on tuna sandwiches is a thing, too (a very good thing, if you ask me). But potato chip cookies are a different thing. There are actual recipes for potato chip cookies. Vintage recipes. As in, your grandmother probably had a recipe for potato chip cookies in her recipe tin. Typically, potato chip cookies fall into the same cookie genre as Mexican wedding cookies or pecan sandies, as in they're kind of dry and crumbly and, often, dusted in confectioners' sugar. But this isn't what I would expect when hearing "potato chip cookies"; the name seems to suggest something other than what they ultimately are. To me, *potato chip cookie* evokes a deliciously sweet and salty treat with chunks of potato chips peeking out of a tender, chewy cookie. So, that's what I set out to invent. This cookie is chewy, sweet and salty, and exactly what a potato chip cookie should be. (Betcha can't eat just one!)

Makes about 3 dozen cookies

½ pound (2 sticks) unsalted butter, at room temperature

1 cup brown sugar

¼ cup granulated sugar

2 teaspoons vanilla extract

2 large eggs

2 cups all-purpose flour

1 teaspoon baking soda

1 teaspoon coarse sea salt

3 cups crushed salted potato chips (kettle, ruffled—it doesn't really matter)

Flaky sea salt

1. Preheat your oven to 375°F and line two or three baking sheets with parchment paper.

2. Place the butter in the bowl of a stand mixer fitted with a paddle attachment, or use a large bowl and an electric hand mixer. Beat for 2 minutes, or until light and fluffy. Add the brown and granulated sugar and mix on medium speed for 3 to 5 minutes. Add the vanilla and eggs and beat until fully incorporated.

3. Beat in the flour, baking soda, and coarse salt on low speed just until combined. Using a wooden spoon, stir in 2 cups of crushed potato chips.

4. Roll the dough into 1½-inch balls and roll them in the remaining cup of crushed potato chips until coated. (If the dough is too sticky to roll in your hands when you start step 4, put it in the fridge for 20 minutes.)

5. Place the balls 2 inches apart on the prepared baking sheets and bake until golden, 11 to 15 minutes. Remove from the oven and let cool on the baking sheets for 5 minutes.

CHERRY-ALMOND OLIVE OIL GRANOLA

I know what you're thinking. *Olive oil in granola?! What's* that *doing in there?* Well, see, the thing about granola—really good granola—is that it needs to be not only sweet and chewy, but also crispy and crunchy. Sure, flavor is important (a balance of sweet and salty, toasty, and a bit fruity is the ideal balance in my book), but what sets a really great granola apart from a so-so batch is getting the texture just right. Olive oil gives granola a crispy, crackly lightness.

Other reasons to love a granola featuring olive oil? There's no melting or heating to make it stirrable—unlike recipes that call for butter or coconut oil—so it naturally lends itself to a speedy dump-stir-bake kind of prep, and who doesn't love *that* brand of simplicity? And, of course, there's the unique fruity, savory, pleasingly bitter quality that only olive oil can deliver and that perfectly complements the recipe's earthy ingredients. All of the nuts, seeds, spices—even the sweetener—are up for grabs here, so tweak the ingredients list to your liking. Use brown sugar in place of maple syrup. Hazelnuts instead of almonds? Sure! Dried pineapple instead of cherries? Go for it. As long as you let the olive oil do its work, you'll be golden.

Makes about 6 cups granola

4 cups rolled oats

1 cup hulled pumpkin seeds

1 cup unsweetened coconut

1¼ cups whole or roughly chopped raw almonds

¼ cup light brown sugar

½ teaspoon ground cinnamon

1 teaspoon coarse sea salt

½ cup extra virgin olive oil

¾ cup pure maple syrup

1 cup dried cherries

1. Preheat the oven to 325°F. Line a rimmed baking sheet with parchment paper.

2. Combine the oats, seeds, coconut, almonds, light brown sugar, cinnamon, and coarse salt in a large bowl. Stir to mix. Add the olive oil and maple syrup and stir until fully incorporated. Spread the mixture in an even layer on the prepared baking sheet.

3. Bake, stirring occasionally, until the granola is golden brown and toasted, 30 to 40 minutes.

4. Remove the granola from the oven and season with more coarse salt to taste. Let cool completely on a wire rack, then stir in the dried cherries.

5. Store in an airtight container for up to 2 months.

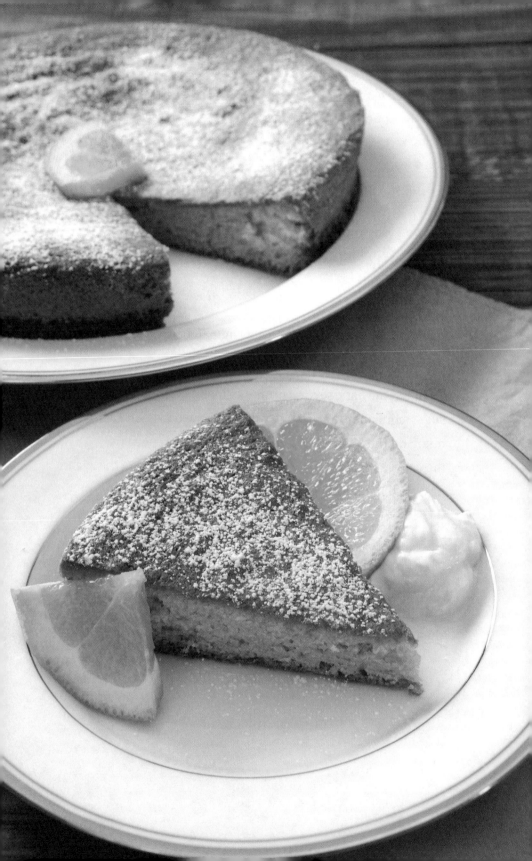

ALMOND OLIVE OIL CAKE

A luscious combination of extra virgin olive oil, almonds, and bright lemon, this cake is exceptionally good—and I say this as a staunch butter-makes-it-better proselyte. Butter-free as this cake may be, it is unbelievably moist and it stays that way, getting even better the longer it sits on the counter. (As if you're even going to have the chance to find that out! It'll be gone before you know it, I promise.) The cake itself is bright and beautiful and can be served with just a dusting of confectioners' sugar. If you want to take things one step further, give the optional brown butter glaze a try for just a bit of richness.

As for the olive oil, its taste plays a starring role here, so use one that's unrefined to get maximum flavor. I like an oil with a peppery bite that will provide a bit of interest and flavor contrast, but it's totally a matter of personal preference—simply stick with something that tastes good to you. Want to take things a step further? Consider an infused olive oil, like lemon, grapefruit, or even basil.

Serves 8 to 10

Continued

Butter, for pan

1 cup all-purpose flour, plus more for dusting

½ cup almond flour

1½ teaspoons baking powder

1 teaspoon coarse sea salt

3 large eggs

¾ cup granulated sugar

½ cup plus 1 tablespoon extra virgin olive oil

½ teaspoon pure vanilla extract

¼ teaspoon pure almond extract

Grated zest of 1 lemon

½ cup fresh orange juice

Confectioners' sugar for dusting (optional)

OPTIONAL GLAZE

2 tablespoons unsalted butter

1 cup confectioners' sugar

3 tablespoons whole milk

1. Preheat the oven to 350°F. Butter and flour a 9-inch round cake pan or springform pan.

2. Whisk together the all-purpose and almond flour, baking powder, and coarse salt in a medium bowl.

3. Combine the eggs and granulated sugar in a separate large bowl. Whisk thoroughly, then add the olive oil, vanilla and almond extracts, lemon zest, and orange juice and beat until the mixture is light yellow, about 1 minute.

4. Slowly add the dry ingredients to the wet, beating until you achieve a smooth batter.

5. Pour the batter into the prepared pan and bake until a cake tester inserted into the center comes out clean, 35 to 45 minutes.

6. Remove from the oven and let the cake cool in the pan for 10 minutes, then remove it from the pan and allow it to cool completely on a rack. Once cool, serve the cake as is, with a dusting of confectioners' sugar or, if you'd like, with the following glaze:

7. Heat the butter in a saucepan over medium heat until golden brown, about 10 minutes. Set aside to cool slightly.

8. While the butter cools, whisk together the confectioners' sugar and milk in a medium bowl. Slowly pour in the butter, whisking to combine. Immediately pour over the cake. Allow the glaze to set, then serve.

OLIVE OIL PUMPKIN BREAD

Did you know that your favorite olive oil is truly great for baking? And not in a "look how cute! That olive oil is trying to be butter!" kind of way. It's actually, on its own, really excellent in all kinds of baked goods. It works for texture, for flavor, and for nutrition—in some cases even more so than butter. For one thing, it's full of vitamins, antioxidants, and healthy fats (but you knew that already). And it tastes fantastic—rich and complex. But what I love about it, especially in instances like this couldn't-be-easier pumpkin bread recipe (and where it's added to muffins, cakes, and brownies), is that it keeps the finished product tender and moist for longer than those made with butter, which dry out after only a couple of days.

This loaf can, technically, hang around on your counter for several days, just improving with age. (If you don't have two little pumpkin-bread-eating monsters living under your roof, as I do, you may get the chance to find out.) It even freezes well and works nicely as muffins. No one's going to arrest you for adding chocolate chips or nuts here. And while I have some strong feelings about raisins in baked goods, playing around with add-ins is generally encouraged.

Makes two 9-by-5-inch loaves

Butter or oil, for pan (optional)

3½ cups all-purpose flour

2 teaspoons baking soda

1½ teaspoons fine sea salt

1 teaspoon ground nutmeg

1 teaspoon ground cinnamon

1 teaspoon ground cloves

1 teaspoon ground ginger

2 cups pure pumpkin puree

3 cups sugar

4 large eggs

1 cup extra virgin olive oil

⅔ cup water

1. Preheat the oven to 350°F and grease two 9-by-5-inch loaf pans and/or line with parchment paper.

2. Combine the flour, baking soda, fine salt, and spices in a medium bowl. Set aside.

3. Combine the pumpkin puree and sugar in a large bowl, beating with an electric hand mixer or whisking until well mixed. Add the eggs and olive oil and beat to incorporate, scraping down the sides of the bowl as needed. With the mixer on low speed, add the flour mixture in two batches, alternating with the water; beat to combine.

4. Divide the batter evenly between the two prepared loaf pans.

5. Bake for about an hour, or until a toothpick inserted in the center of the loaf comes out clean. Transfer to a wire rack to cool for 10 minutes. Turn out of the pans and let cool completely.

OLIVE OIL CHOCOLATE MOUSSE

Lest you think I'm just an absolute glutton, with not just one, but three recipes in this book that combine olive oil and chocolate, allow me to point out that a recent study published by the European Society of Cardiology showed that the combination of chocolate and olive oil in small portions may improve your cardiovascular risk profile. So, really, what we're talking about here is some straight-up health food. (Okay, maybe not quite, but still . . .)

Sure, this recipe probably slants a bit more toward "treat" than anything else, but it is undeniably delicious, decadently rich, and very simple to make. Based on a Spanish version of chocolate mousse, with extra virgin olive oil standing in for the usual heavy cream, this mousse is velvety smooth with just a hint of the oil's fruity and subtly savory flavor. Use a mild-tasting oil to let the taste of the chocolate shine through.

Serves 6

6 ounces bittersweet chocolate (preferably 70% cacao), roughly chopped

3 large eggs, separated

⅔ cup confectioners' sugar, sifted after measuring

2 tablespoons prepared espresso or very strong coffee, at room temperature

1 teaspoon Chambord, Cointreau, or Grand Marnier (optional)

¾ cup extra virgin olive oil

Raspberries for garnish (optional)

1. Microwave the chocolate in a small microwave-safe bowl or in a saucepan over very low heat, until melted. Let cool to lukewarm.

Continued

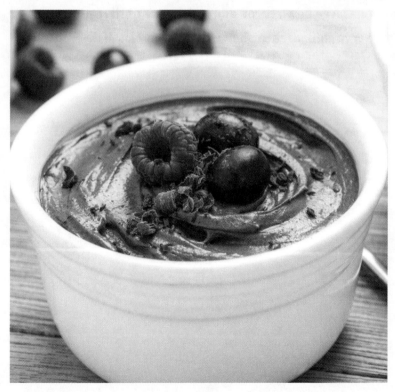

2. Combine the egg yolks and confectioners' sugar in the bowl of a stand mixer fitted with the whisk attachment, or use a large bowl and an electric hand mixer. Beat the egg yolks and sugar on medium speed until smooth. Add the coffee and liqueur (if using) and beat to combine. Mix in the melted chocolate and the olive oil and mix well.

3. Whip the egg whites in a separate medium bowl until stiff peaks form. Fold the beaten egg whites into the chocolate mixture, one-third at a time, thoroughly combining in between additions until all the whites have been folded in. Do not overmix.

4. Spoon the mixture into six to eight individual ramekins or one large bowl, cover, and refrigerate until ready to eat. Serve chilled, garnished with raspberries, if desired.

RICH OLIVE OIL BROWNIES WITH FLAKED SALT

If you want to know the key to my heart, it's brownies. Moist, fudgy, and intensely chocolaty. That's my cure for a bad day. These brownies, rich with two kinds of chocolate and the subtle caramel flavor of brown sugar, come together in no time and yield a deep, dense, uncomplicated bake. It's about as classic a brownie recipe as you can find with two small departures: the olive oil, of course, and the shower of flaky salt on top. The oil lends an understated richness and ever-so-slight fruitiness to the brownie, and the extra salt not only balances the sweetness and punches up their chocolatiness, but adds a welcome crunch to each bite.

So, that's all well and good, but I'll let you in on a tip that just might blow your mind, one that I learned from a California olive oil producer who serves olive oil brownies in her tasting room: make these brownies with flavored olive oil. Tangerine olive oil, jalapeño olive oil, anything you can find that suits your fancy. Either way—classic or tricked out—these brownies are pretty darn perfect.

Makes about 16 brownies

Continued

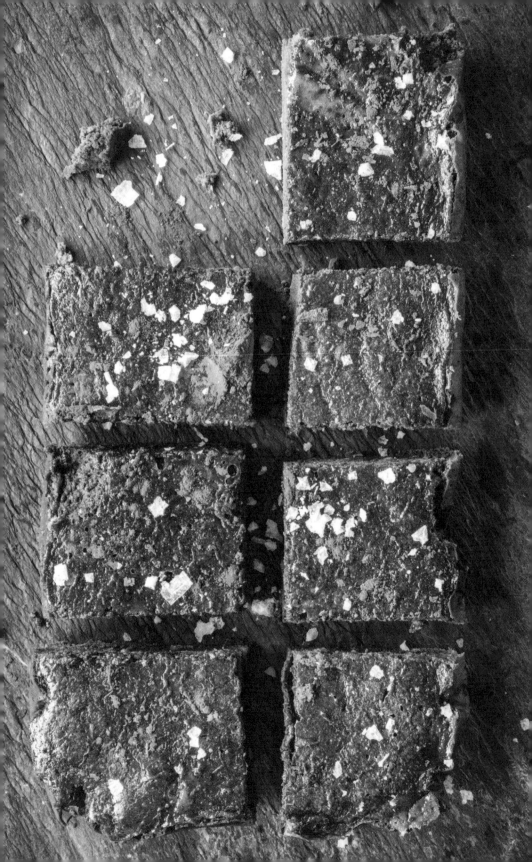

Olive oil, for pan

1 cup all-purpose flour

¼ cup Dutch-processed cocoa powder

¾ teaspoon coarse sea salt

¼ teaspoon baking powder

⅓ cup mild extra virgin olive oil

4 ounces melted semisweet or bittersweet chocolate

1 large egg, at room temperature

1 tablespoon vanilla extract

¾ cup packed dark brown sugar

¼ cup granulated sugar

½ cup chocolate chips

Flaky sea salt, such as Maldon

1. Preheat the oven to 350°F. Brush an 8-inch square baking pan with the oil. Line with parchment paper, leaving an overhang on two opposite sides for easy removal.

2. Whisk together flour, cocoa powder, coarse salt, and baking powder in a medium bowl. Set aside.

3. Whisk together the olive oil, melted chocolate, egg, and vanilla in a large bowl. Add the brown and granulated sugar, whisking until smooth.

4. Fold in the flour mixture and chocolate chips. Pour the batter into the prepared pan. Bake until a toothpick comes out clean, 20 to 25 minutes. Remove from the oven and, while still hot, sprinkle with flaky salt. Let cool completely on a wire rack. To serve, cut into 2-inch squares.

EASY AS PIE OLIVE OIL TART CRUST

Making traditional piecrust—the kind with butter and chilling and rolling with a rolling pin—is *really* not difficult. Pie dough has earned a bad rap in that respect and I'm here to tell you that it is nothing to be afraid of. That said, there is certainly some effort required and—even harder to come by some days—some semblance of patience involved in making pie dough from scratch.

For days when you want to knock out a pie or a tart and you just can't face even the slightest hassle, it really doesn't get easier than this five-ingredient olive oil tart dough. It's pressed into the tart pan, so there's no rolling. The dough is ready to work with as soon as you make it, so there's no chilling or resting required—and no hassle. It works for both sweet and savory applications (simply omit the sugar for the latter) and, if you're vegan, you can replace the whole milk with plant-based milk or even water.

Makes one 10-inch tart crust or piecrust

1½ cups plus 2 tablespoons all-purpose flour

¾ teaspoon coarse sea salt

1 teaspoon sugar (optional)

½ cup mild olive oil

2 tablespoons whole milk

1. Stir together the flour, ½ teaspoon of the coarse salt, and the sugar (if using) in a medium bowl.

2. Whisk together the olive oil and milk in a small bowl.

3. Combine wet and dry ingredients, mixing gently with a fork, just until mixed.

4. Transfer the dough to a 10-inch tart or pie pan and pat out the dough, pressing gently with your hands so that it covers the bottom and sides of the pan.

5. The dough is now ready to use with your favorite tart or pie recipe!

Note: To blind-bake, prick the unbaked crust all over with a fork. Preheat the oven to 350°F, then bake the crust for 15 minutes, or until lightly golden. You can then fill the tart shell and bake the tart again for another 20 to 40 minutes, depending on the filling.

HEALING
TREATMENTS

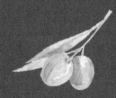

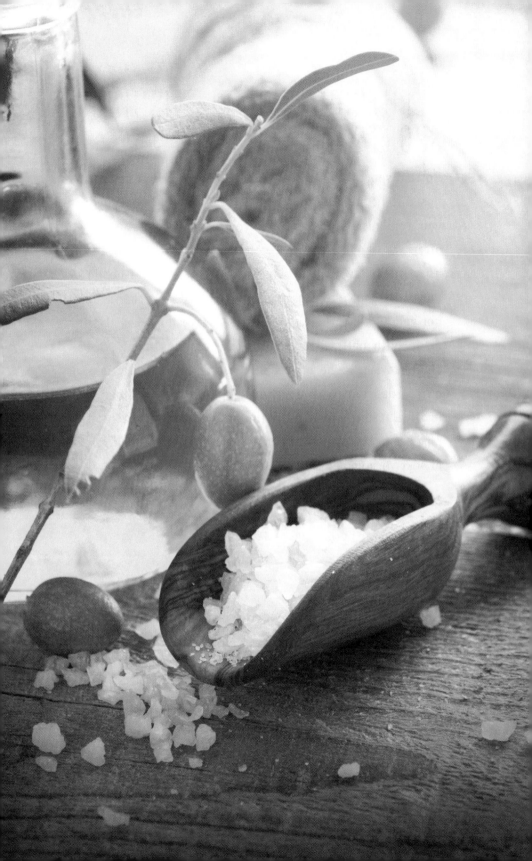

ELECTROLYTE-REPLENISHING SPORTS DRINK

Bottled sports drinks are a real head-scratcher. They're supposed to be good for you, right? They're supposed to hydrate you, replenish fluids and electrolytes, and help you recover after a workout. But they're often loaded with sugar as well as artificial flavors and color. I mean, they're neon—need I say more? My choice for postworkout renewal is neither red #40 nor yellow #6; rather, it's this super refreshing herbal drink, made with naturally occurring electrolytes from sea salt. Make it with the herbal tea of your choice; my go-to is mint, but it's delicious with anything from hibiscus to lemon, even licorice. It keeps for a long time in the fridge, so feel free to make a huge pitcher and keep it at the ready for a week's worth of postworkout refresh.

Makes 1 quart sports drink

4 cups brewed herbal tea, cooled

2 to 4 tablespoons raw honey or pure maple syrup

¼ teaspoon fine sea salt

1. Combine all the ingredients in a large bottle or pitcher. Stir or shake well.

2. Store in the refrigerator for up to 2 weeks.

HANGOVER PREVENTER

I think it's fair to say that no one enjoys a hangover. The headache, nausea, and general everything-hurts sensation is miserable. The best way to avoid a hangover? Not drinking in the first place! Moderation is second best. Better still? Planning ahead to minimize the afterburn when you know cocktails are in your future.

One trick is to try to slow the rate at which your body processes alcohol; olive oil may help with that. Your body metabolizes a serving of alcohol (a glass of wine, a beer, a shot) in 60 to 75 minutes. The faster you drink, the faster your blood alcohol levels rise, which is when you start to dive into prime hangover territory. Taking olive oil before your first drink may slow the rate of absorption, which may give your body time to adjust to its new blood chemistry. Add a bit of alkalizing lemon juice to your pregame and you'll help balance the acidity that alcohol brings into your system. Then add some cinnamon, which mostly just tastes good. With this combo, you may have a better chance of enjoying yourself without having to pay so dearly for it the next day (although you could also just make sure to eat a lot of fatty foods before or while drinking). And, hopefully it goes without saying, but . . . please drink responsibly.

Makes 1 treatment

1 ounce fresh lemon juice

1 ounce cold-pressed virgin olive oil

⅛ teaspoon ground cinnamon

Combine all the ingredients in a small glass. Mix thoroughly, then down the hatch!

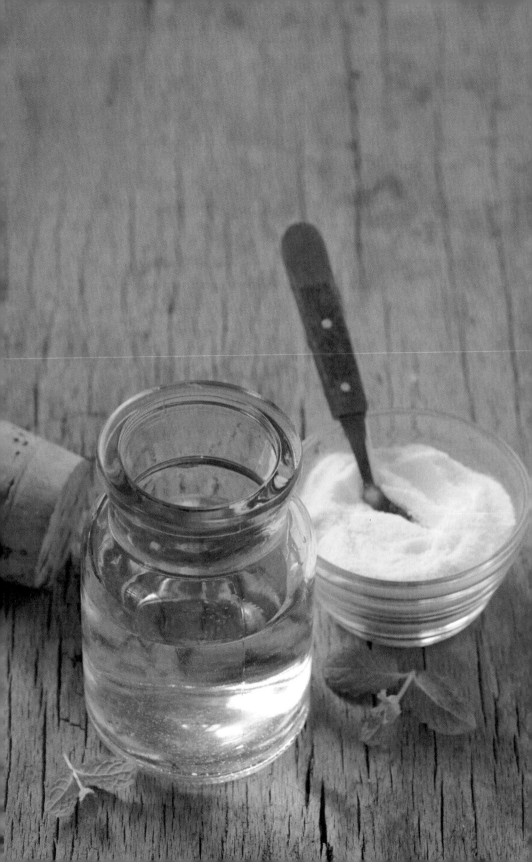

SORE THROAT SOOTHER

There's nothing quite like autumn where I live. There's a chill in the air, apples are ripe for the picking, the leaves turn . . . and every single member of my family manages to begin coughing and sneezing all over each other. Ew. Fall commences with a sore throat and not, as it turns out, with pumpkin spice lattes. To prepare for the inevitable, I keep a healthy stock of fine sea salt on hand for the best, quickest sore throat remedy I know: a saltwater gargle.

It's simple—gargling with warm salt water draws excess fluid from inflamed tissue, which makes it hurt less. It also helps kill bacteria, loosen thick mucus, and remove irritants that make throats hurt. It won't *cure* a sore throat, sorry, but this gargle will definitely relieve pain and inflammation. Bottoms up!

Makes 1 treatment

¼ teaspoon fine sea salt
½ cup warm water

1. Combine the fine salt and warm water in a glass. Stir to dissolve the salt.

2. To use: Gargle for 30 seconds, then spit the solution into the sink. Repeat 3 or 4 times daily.

OLIVE OIL COUGH REMEDY

Being sick stinks. Of all the symptoms that go along with cold and flu season, the one that I dread most is the cough. I've got no patience for it! So, when I'm up against a nagging cough, I lean on this quick home remedy for relief. Olive oil naturally coats your throat, increasing lubrication and reducing the urge to cough. What's more, it reduces inflammation in your throat, much the same way that ibuprofen works, thanks to the anti-inflammatory agent oleocanthal, which is present in both olive oil and ibuprofen. Straight-up olive oil by the spoonful will do the trick to tame a pesky cough. But you can also pump up the volume on the antibacterial and anti-inflammatory beat with this quick and easy homemade cough syrup that combines olive oil with soothing honey and vitamin C–rich lemon.

Makes about 16 doses

¼ cup fresh lemon juice
¼ cup raw honey
½ cup extra virgin olive oil

1. Combine the lemon juice and honey in a small jar or other lidded container.

2. Heat the olive oil in a microwave or on the stovetop just until warm.

3. Add the olive oil to the honey mixture and stir or shake to combine. Store, covered, at room temperature.

4. To use: Take 1 tablespoon every 2 to 3 hours, as needed.

EARACHE RELIEF

It's 4:45 p.m. On a Friday. (Always on a Friday.) And you start to put the pieces together. Your little one has been cranky all afternoon, making it really hard for you to get all of this organizing and packing done. And now she's hanging on to your leg, tugging her ear, and screaming. And it hits you: ear infection! Of course, by the time you realize this, it's too late to get to the pediatrician. But what can you do? You won't be able to see a doctor until the morning, which is when you were supposed to leave town. Well, for now you can treat the pain until a doctor can assess whether your kiddo will need antibiotics. In the meantime, your little one is miserable and you want to know what you can do to make that heartbreaking screaming stop! Try this warm salt sock trick—it'll create a shift in the pressure within the ear, draw out fluid, and ease their discomfort.

Makes 1 reusable compress

1 clean, cotton knee-length sock
1 to 1½ cups coarse sea salt

1. Pour the coarse salt into the sock and tie a knot at the end.

2. Heat the sock in a clean, dry skillet over medium-low heat for 4 to 6 minutes, shaking and/or flipping it every 30 to 60 seconds, until very warm to the touch.

3. Place the warm salt sock over the ear and the area behind the adjacent jawbone. Repeat as needed.

DIY SALINE NOSE SPRAY

Whether resulting from nasal allergies, an infection, or a nasty cold, sinus congestion is really uncomfortable. Using chemical nasal sprays can provide temporary relief, but often comes with side effects and shouldn't be used long term. One of the best alternatives to chemical nasal sprays is saltwater irrigation, which has been shown to decrease the swelling caused by nasal irritants, improve allergy symptoms, and shorten the duration of sinus infections. Regular use may even prevent recurring sinusitis!

Because sinus infections frequently occur when swelling from irritants, allergens, or viruses block the opening of the sinuses, properly aerating and draining them can make a big difference. One of the best ways to do so is with salt water, which can wash away allergens, mucus, and other debris; help to moisten the mucous membranes, and prevent bacteria from growing. Just be sure to use distilled (or previously boiled and cooled) water, to prevent risk of a serious infection from bacteria. Then squirt, sniff, and rinse away, using a bulb syringe or a neti pot.

Makes about 1 cup saline spray

8 ounces distilled, sterile, or boiled and cooled water

½ teaspoon fine sea salt

½ teaspoon baking soda

1. Combine the water, fine salt, and baking soda in a small bowl or jar. Store, covered, at room temperature.

2. To use: Fill a bulb syringe or neti pot with the solution. Stand over a sink and lean your head forward, tilting it to one side. Pour the solution into one nostril, aiming the stream toward the back of your head. The solution will go into your nasal cavity and run out the other nostril. Adjust the position of your head to keep it from running down the back of your throat. Gently blow your nose and spit out the drainage to clear the nasal passages and throat.

3. Repeat with your other nostril.

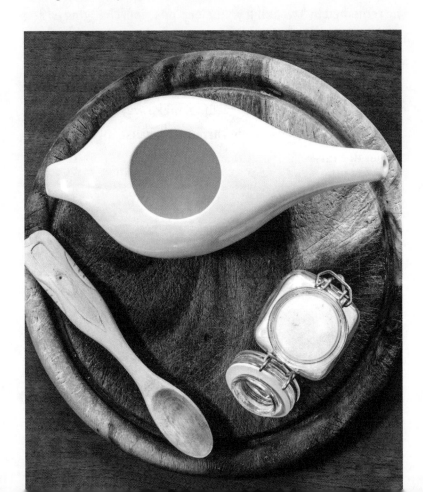

SNORE SOOTHER

Snoring can seriously mess with your sleep quality (or your partner's). And did you know that 25 percent of adults are snorers? Many snorers don't even know it unless their partner tells them (or, you know, smacks them in the middle of the night). When we sleep, the muscles of the throat relax, the tongue falls backward, and the throat becomes narrow and kind of floppy. As we breathe, the walls of the throat actually vibrate, which leads to snoring. The narrower the airway, the louder the snoring.

Most of the time, snoring is harmless—if annoying—and can be remedied by tweaking your sleep position, changing eating and drinking habits, creating a healthy bedtime routine, and relying on a bit of olive oil to quiet things down. A strong anti-inflammatory agent, olive oil eases the tissues along the respiratory passages to reduce swelling, make way for airflow, and lessen the vibrations in the throat that cause all that racket. Sweet dreams!

Makes 1 treatment

½ to 1 teaspoon extra virgin olive oil

Take two or three sips of olive oil before going to bed daily.

Note: Loud, frequent snoring can be a symptom of obstructive sleep apnea, a condition that causes repeated interruptions in breathing. You need to seek out professional treatment for sleep apnea.

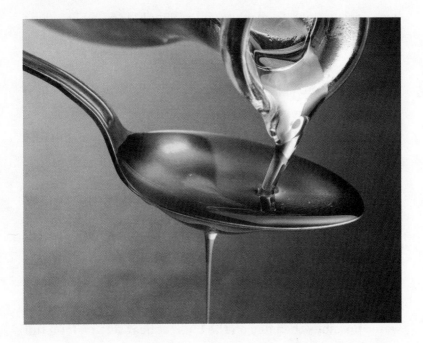

LICE TREATMENT

Lice. The word alone makes my head itch! While we're all susceptible, little kids get lice most often (at a rate of 6 million per year) because they like to be in no-such-thing-as personal-space close contact with each other during playdates, slumber parties, sports activities, and the like. If you've got a school-age kid, trust me, you're going to want to have this remedy in your back pocket. Now, if and when you or your kids do get lice, don't panic. (I've tried panicking—it doesn't get rid of lice.) Instead, grab the nearest bottle of olive oil and get dousing.

Why olive oil? It both suffocates the active lice (live ones) and makes it easier to remove nits (eggs), although it will not kill them. Plus it's not full of pesticides, which—let's agree—are almost as scary as an out-of-control case of lice. Just remember, delousing an infested head is only part of the battle. Other steps to ensure you rid your life of lice: place brushes, combs, ponytail holders, and other hair accessories in a resealable plastic bag and place in the freezer for 24 hours; wash and dry all bedding, clothing that has been worn by those affected, stuffed animals, and towels in the hottest water possible, then dry on the highest heat setting for a full cycle plus an extra 20 minutes; and thoroughly wipe down and vacuum car headrests and seats.

Makes 1 treatment

Olive oil (amount will vary depending on hair length)

1. Blow dry hair, section by section, using as hot a setting as can be tolerated, for 15 to 20 minutes. (Lice can't survive high temperatures.)

2. Apply olive oil to the hair and scalp, using enough to thoroughly and evenly saturate. To protect clothing and furniture, you may want to cover the hair with a plastic shower cap afterward. Allow the olive oil to remain on the hair for at least 8 hours.

3. Using a metal lice comb (a very fine-toothed comb), work section by section to remove the nits (tiny white nubs clinging to the hair shaft), wiping the comb with a paper towel as you go. Repeat until no more lice appear on the paper towel.

4. Wash the hair to remove olive oil with a gentle shampoo, then blow dry again.

5. Continue to comb the hair daily with the fine comb until all nits have been removed.

OLIVE OIL AND SEA SALT BATH FOR ITCHY, IRRITATED SKIN

Dry air, cold weather, sun, age, even stress and anxiety, can cause dry, itchy skin. More often than not, inflamed, uncomfortable, scaly, or cracked skin from these causes isn't serious, but it *can* be a real pain—literally! One surefire way to relieve discomfort is to soak in an olive oil and sea salt bath. With anti-inflammatory and antioxidant compounds—thanks in large part to something called oleocanthal—extra virgin olive oil can trigger a variety of biological reactions that are necessary for wound healing and skin repair, such as cell migration, cell proliferation, and new tissue growth. And, of course, it's just a great moisturizer that feels good on your skin.

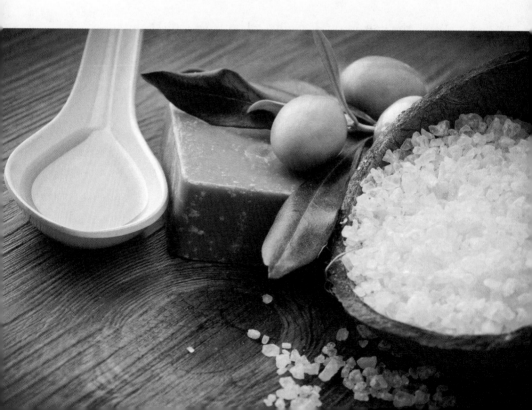

Meanwhile, sea salt helps remove scales and decreases the bothersome itching caused by such conditions as eczema, psoriasis, dehydration, and acne. And sea salt's mineral content helps restore the protective barrier in skin, which helps it hold hydration. When added to a warm bath, olive oil and sea salt provide all-over relief for uncomfortable skin. Just keep an eye on the temperature of your bath—water that's too hot can actually make dry skin worse. So, make sure you're erring on the side of warm rather than hot and you'll be in great shape.

Makes 1 treatment

¼ cup extra virgin olive oil

¼ cup sea salt

1. Fill a bathtub with enough warm water to completely submerge yourself, adding the olive oil and sea salt as the tub fills.

2. Submerge yourself and soak for 10 to 15 minutes.

3. Repeat as needed.

BUG BITE SOOTHER

My family loves an outdoor movie night on the porch! Except for one, incessantly annoying, relentless thing. The mosquitoes! We're usually all eaten alive and wake up an itchy mess the next morning. So to soothe our bites, I reach for one of the surest remedies I know: sea salt.

It might sound like we literally add salt to our wounds, I know, but here's the thing: mosquito bites itch and swell because our cells release histamine, a compound that signals infection-fighting white blood cells to get to work, when mosquito saliva (a foreign body) enters our bloodstream. The blood flow causes redness and swelling around the bite and causes the nerves in the area to itch. Sea salt counteracts this swelling and itching, thanks to its antiseptic and anti-inflammatory properties. So, next time you're out on a summer night without bug spray, keep the sea salt close by.

Makes 1 treatment

1 teaspoon fine sea salt
A few drops of water

1. Combine the fine salt with enough water to make a paste.

2. Spread it on the affected area.

3. Allow the paste to remain on the skin for 10 to 30 minutes. Rinse with cool water.

SUNBURN SOOTHER

Long beachy vacations, afternoons lounging by the pool, and lazy walks in the summer sun . . . all the hallmarks of a perfect summer day are also some of the best ways to end up with a first-class sunburn. Sure, we do our best to prevent them—we slather on sunscreen, try to avoid midday sun, and seek shade when we can, but occasionally we slip up and then . . . whomp whomp: damage done. If you do end up with a burn despite your best efforts, you can actually ease the pain and discomfort with olive oil. Its antioxidant properties protect skin cells against environmental damage, inflammation, and irritation, which means it'll provide pain relief. And because olive oil is also super moisturizing, it's a godsend for parched, sunburned skin. One word of warning: Don't put oil on your skin if you're going back into the sun anytime soon. Just think about what happens to an egg in a pan of hot oil . . .

Makes 1 treatment

Extra virgin olive oil

Liberally rub a coating of olive oil on the affected area, gently massaging it so that the oil penetrates the skin. Repeat twice daily until the condition improves.

POISON IVY RELIEF

Ever hear the saying "Leaves of three, let it be"? Yep, we all know the drill: when you're out in nature, step away from the poison ivy or else learn the hard way and pack your bags for Itchy City. Urushiol—the oily substance on poison ivy that causes a rash—can bond to the skin (and clothes and gardening tools) in about a minute. And if, like 85 percent of the population, you're allergic to urushiol, you'll be facing an itchy, oozing rash in a heartbeat. The good news, if there is any, is that a poison ivy reaction is not contagious. Super uncomfortable, yes. But not contagious. It can, however, spread on your body, so if you know you've come into contact with poison ivy, wash your skin and clothes right away. You can treat a mild case of poison ivy rash at home with this cooling, soothing salt treatment, inspired by an old-school farmers' almanac remedy.

Makes 1 treatment

1 tablespoon fine sea salt

⅛ teaspoon peppermint essential oil

1 to 2 cups green clay

A few teaspoons of water

1. Combine the fine salt, peppermint oil, and clay with enough water to achieve a thick but spreadable paste.

2. Apply liberally to the affected area and leave in place for approximately 30 minutes. Rinse thoroughly with warm water. Gently pat dry.

3. Repeat two or three times daily.

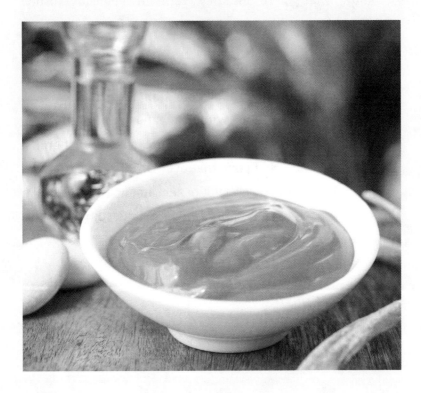

JELLYFISH STING TREATMENT

A day at the beach. There's nothing like it. The splashing and jumping, dunking and diving beneath the waves. When all of a sudden . . . hot, shooting pain on your skin? Yep, you've been stung by a jellyfish and, holy moly, does it hurt. But is it any wonder? A bee sting leaves behind a single stinger that you can usually see and pull out; when a jellyfish stings, it leaves thousands of tiny little stingers that continue to release jellyfish venom into the person's body even after they're detached from the jelly. The burn is . . . beyond.

I know what you're thinking. We've all seen that episode of *Friends*. But after you're stung, you actually shouldn't pee on it. Urine doesn't help the sting. (Thank goodness, because *ick*.) So what does work? Well, first you'll need to use tweezers to pull off any tentacles still on your skin. After that, experts agree that rinsing the sting with salt water is one of the most effective ways to relieve discomfort. Sure, you can just grab a bucket of seawater and pour that over the affected area, but you need to be really careful not to get sand or other debris in the sting. A better, safer approach is to make your own salt-water solution that is about 3.5 percent salinity—just like the ocean—like so:

Makes 1 treatment

3½ teaspoons fine sea salt

4½ cups clean, cool tap water

1. Combine the fine salt and cool water in a pitcher or large bowl. Stir to combine.

2. Rinse the affected area with the salt water.

3. Gently pat dry with a soft towel or cloth. Repeat as necessary.

Note: Any of the following symptoms constitute a medical emergency. Call 911 immediately if the person who has been stung:

- has trouble breathing or swallowing
- has a swollen tongue or lips, or a change in voice
- feels nauseated or is vomiting
- is dizzy or has a headache
- has muscle spasms
- has stings over a large part of the body
- was stung in the eye or mouth
- may have been stung by a very dangerous type of jellyfish

SOOTHING FOOT SOAK

Whether you've spent a workday standing on hard surfaces, hoofed it for hours on a sightseeing tour, hiked for miles in the woods, or stood for longer than you care to admit waiting in amusement park lines with two children who seem to have eaten Energizer batteries for breakfast, chances are you aren't a complete stranger to tired, achy feet. The good news is that relief for tired tootsies is a quick soak away. With olive oil for moisture, sea salt for reducing swelling and inflammation, and peppermint for a soothing and cooling effect, this soak couldn't be easier to prepare. And it's not only relaxing, it's a great way to get some vitamins and nutrients back into your skin, because your feet don't get a day off. You'll be up and at 'em again tomorrow!

Makes 1 treatment

2 tablespoons coarse sea salt

¼ cup olive oil

5 to 8 drops peppermint essential oil

1. Combine the coarse salt, olive oil, and peppermint oil in a foot bath or basin large enough to accommodate your feet.

2. Add enough warm water to cover your feet.

3. Relax and soak for 15 to 20 minutes.

CRACKED HEEL TREATMENT

Putting your best foot forward may seem like an impossibility if you suffer from cracked heels. Forget cute—dry, cracked heels are more than just an eyesore—they're a *sore* sore! And because the skin in the heel area is thicker and tougher than on other parts of the body, treating it requires a bit more effort. You can't just slap on some lotion and call it a day. One of the best ways to soften and moisturize cracked heels is with this soak. White vinegar works to disinfect the skin and—bonus!—treat odors, while olive oil sinks deep into the heels to create a natural moisture barrier. Sure it might smell like salad dressing, but it really does work. And I can assure you, no one will swing by your table, asking, "Would you like freshly ground pepper?"

Makes 1 treatment

¼ cup olive oil
½ cup white vinegar
Warm water

1. Combine the olive oil and vinegar in a basin large enough to accommodate your feet. Add enough warm water to cover your feet. Relax and soak for 10 to 15 minutes.

2. Remove your feet from the mixture and, if you like, gently exfoliate using a pumice stone or scrub (page 204) before drying and moisturizing.

Note: If the cracks on your heels are very deep or become infected, you should see a podiatrist.

INGROWN TOENAIL TREATMENT

Fortunately, an angry, throbbing ingrown toenail is usually not serious and fairly easy to fix with sea salt playing the role of hero. Because an ingrown nail occurs when a sharp corner of the nail digs into the skin at the end of (or on the side of) the toe, you need to free and redirect that portion of the nail to find relief and to prevent infection. Soaking the affected foot in warm salt water will reduce inflammation and help soften the skin so that the nail can grow back properly.

Makes 1 treatment

1 quart warm water

2 tablespoons coarse sea salt

1. Combine the warm water and coarse salt in a large basin or bucket. Stir well to dissolve.

2. Soak the affected foot for 15 to 20 minutes.

3. Gently pat dry with a clean towel. Repeat two or three times a day until the swelling and pain subside.

Note: If the toe doesn't get better in a week or so and/or if infection appears to have set in, see a doctor.

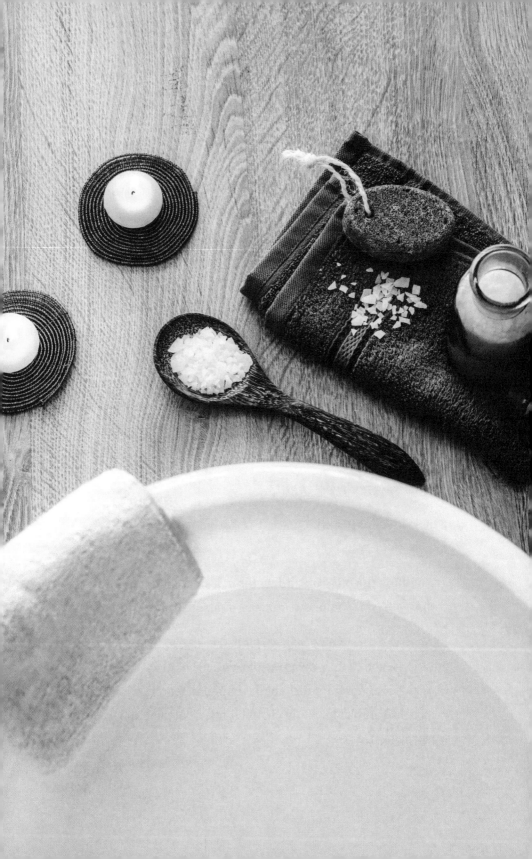

DIAPER RASH SOOTHER

I used to sit and stare at my kids when they were babies and marvel at their skin. Poreless; smooth as silk; and soft as, well, soft as a baby's bottom. And that's ironic, isn't it? Because what's the one part of a baby that is often *not* soft, smooth, and blemish-free? Yep, their bottom. And diaper rash is usually the culprit—puffy and warm with small, uncomfortable bumps all over that little bottom and thighs. Ouch! Poor baby! But there's no reason to worry! Diaper rash is totally treatable and normally goes away in a matter of days if cared for properly. One approach that works really well is to use an olive oil emulsion such as the one here, to not only moisturize and soothe your little one's irritated skin but also to prevent future flare-ups. Mix the emulsion directly in a spray bottle and stash it in your diaper bag for a handy on-the-go treatment.

Makes several treatments

2 tablespoons olive oil
1 tablespoon water

1. Combine the olive oil and water in a small lidded jar or spray bottle. Shake the mixture vigorously.

2. To use: After you've gently cleaned and dried your baby's skin (when diaper rash is really raging, skip the baby wipes and opt for cotton balls dipped in water), apply the olive oil emulsion, using clean hands, a cotton ball, or a spray bottle.

NATURAL LAXATIVE

Constipation. Whether from medication, hormones, a poor diet, lack of exercise, stress, or one of the many other causes of constipation, there's no arguing that it is uncomfortable, unfun, and a literal pain in the you-know-what. And while a pound of prevention (namely in the form of plenty of fiber and water intake, regular exercise, and stress management) is worth a pound of cure, the fact of the matter is that sometimes you just need to feel better ASAP. That's when olive oil swoops in to save the day. It's nutrient-dense and, as such, stimulates the digestive system. It also lubricates the bowels and provides antioxidant protection at the same time. So, in other words, olive oil will get things moving when you're a little backed up. Here's how.

Makes 1 treatment

1 tablespoon extra virgin olive oil

Take the tablespoon of olive oil on an empty stomach, ideally before eating breakfast in the morning.

Note: If olive oil doesn't help get things moving, or if you find that you're chronically constipated, talk to your doctor. In some cases, chronic constipation can be caused by another underlying health condition.

BEAUTY SECRETS

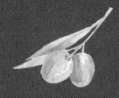

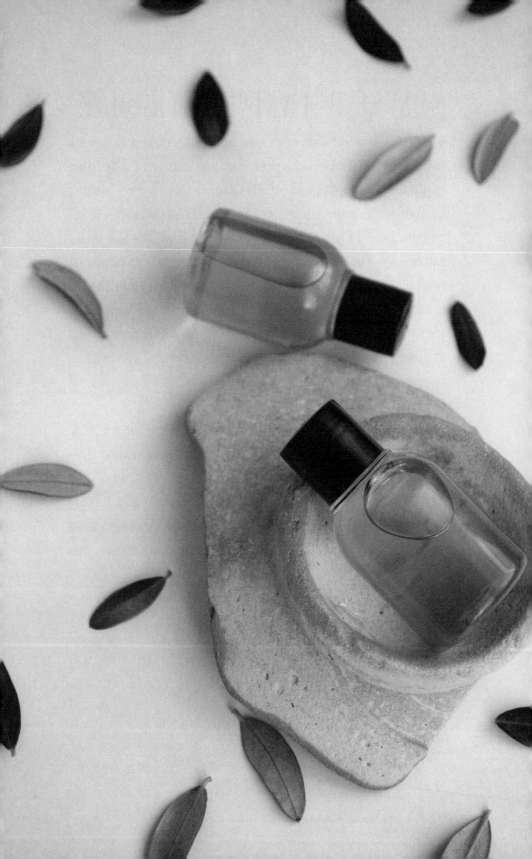

MUSCLE-RELAXING BATH SOAK

There are few indulgences more luxurious than a long soak in a warm tub. I do take baths from time to time and find that while simply slipping into a tub full of warm water is soothing enough on its own, adding sea salt is definitely the quickest and easiest way to take a bath to the next level. For one thing, salt is a great muscle relaxant—particularly great if you've just pushed through a killer CrossFit session or sweaty run. In fact, clinically speaking, there is evidence that salt is beneficial in treating a variety of rheumatic diseases, including rheumatoid arthritis, psoriatic arthritis, and knee osteoarthritis. In addition, sea salt brings anti-inflammatory relief to your whole system.

Although salt on its own makes for a lovely, soothing bath, I do like to toss in a few other ingredients to boost the relaxation and restorative properties, but nothing too crazy—just Epsom salts for an additional hit of magnesium and baking soda for its skin-soothing properties. And if I happen to have some essential oils on hand, I'll toss those in, too.

Makes about 4 treatments

1 cup Epsom salts

1 cup coarse sea salt

½ cup baking soda

2 tablespoons neutral carrier oil, such as grapeseed or sesame

20 drops essential oil (I like lavender, bergamot, rose, or
   chamomile for relaxation, but use what you like)

1. Combine the Epsom salts, coarse salt, and baking soda in a
   small bowl.

2. Add the oils and stir until fully incorporated, breaking up
   any clumps.

3. Store in a lidded container in a cool, dark place. Use ½ to
   1 cup per bath.

MOISTURIZING BODY EXFOLIATOR

Would it be weird for me to call this body scrub delicious? Because it is—decadent and delicious. It's a luxurious combination of salt and olive oil that smooths and moisturizes. It's loaded with vitamins and minerals that actually replenish and nourish from the outside in. And it does wonders for skin that's out of balance, because olive oil and sea salt both help boost hydration, strengthen the skin's moisture barrier, and kickstart the cell-to-cell communication that slows down with age.

When you make this scrub, feel free to customize it with additional skin-nourishing ingredients, such as soothing aloe vera, redness-reducing lavender, or healing carrot-seed essential oil. And when choosing which salt to use, always opt for fine sea salt, as the coarse stuff is abrasive and should be reserved only for rough and tough areas, such as heels and elbows. I highly recommend Dead Sea salt, as it is one of the most nutrient-rich salts on the planet. You can also opt for the readily available Himalayan pink salt or black lava salt, which has the added benefit of cleansing and toxin-removing activated charcoal. Of course, you can always splurge on fancy scrubs that have other "powerful" ingredients, but crafting your own bespoke blend that boosts circulation, exfoliates dead skin, and improves the overall look and feel of your body's largest organ—for a fraction of the price—is pretty darn satisfying.

Makes about 1 cup exfoliator

1 cup fine sea salt

⅓ cup extra virgin olive oil

15 drops essential oil (rosehip, carrot seed, or any oil you have on hand; optional)

1 teaspoon dried lavender buds (optional)

1. Combine the fine salt and olive oil in a small bowl. Stir well.

2. Add the essential oil and/or lavender (if using). Mix again.

3. Store in a lidded container in a cool, dark place for up to 1 year.

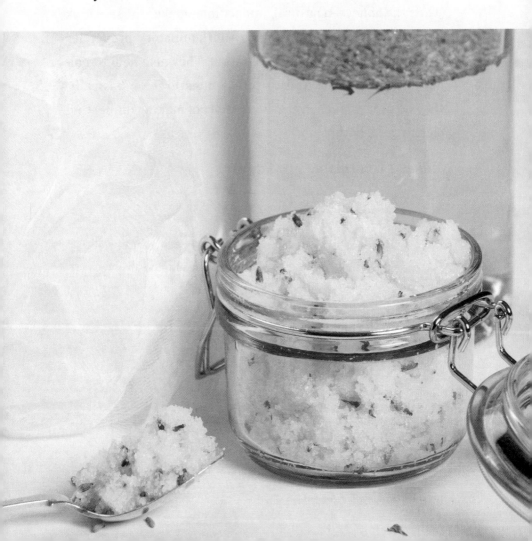

BALANCING FACIAL MASK

Here's a simple at-home mask that gently exfoliates, calms inflammation, and plumps the skin with some much-needed hydration, all in one fell swoop—hockey pros, correct me if I'm wrong, but I believe that's what you refer to as a "hat trick" in the biz. Salt and honey—two powerful skin allies—work together here to balance, protect, and restore your complexion, leaving you with fresh, glowing skin. Salt, a gentle exfoliant, sloughs dead skin cells and improves texture, while the honey—a natural humectant—makes the skin look plump and dewy. Both bring anti-inflammatory properties to soothe skin and to calm irritation. They also help to balance oil production and to retain moisture. So, basically, they do pretty much everything, short of making dinner and cleaning the bathroom.

Makes 1 treatment

2 teaspoons fine sea salt

1 tablespoon raw honey

1. Combine the fine salt and honey in a small bowl. Stir well.

2. To use: Apply the mixture evenly to clean, dry skin, avoiding the eye area. Leave on the skin for 10 to 15 minutes. Using your fingers, rub gently in a circular motion to exfoliate the skin, then rinse thoroughly with warm water.

3. Follow with your usual skin-care routine.

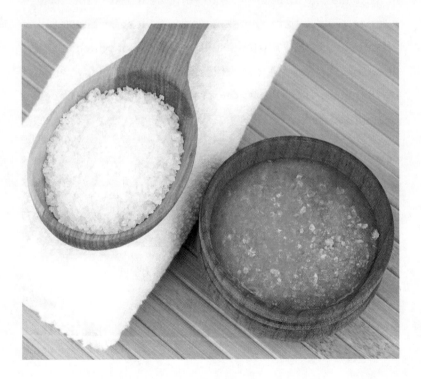

AGE-DEFYING FACIAL SCRUB

It must be the kid in me, but I never tire of putting food on my face. I always feel that I'm getting away with something, somehow breaking the rules. It's so fun! This (entirely edible) homemade face scrub nourishes skin with powerful antioxidants that zap harmful free radicals. And that's not all—it is full of acids that unclog pores and clear out old, dead skin; minerals (such as calcium, magnesium, and potassium) that help moisturize and firm skin; and—in true age-defying style—lycopene, which improves skin elasticity. It's also chock-full of vitamins A, C, and K (thanks, olive oil), all of which contribute to healthy skin. With nothing more than salt, olive oil, and fresh tomato, this all-natural scrub is so good you might even be tempted to eat it!

Makes about ½ cup scrub

¼ cup fine sea salt

2 tablespoons extra virgin olive oil

2 tablespoons finely diced tomato

1. Combine the fine salt and olive oil in a bowl and stir until just mixed.

2. Add the tomato and muddle the mixture together until just incorporated.

3. Store in a lidded container and refrigerate for up to 2 weeks.

EYE DEPUFFER

Some mornings are rougher than others. You know the ones I'm talking about. You wake up, stagger to the bathroom, and come face-to-face with some seriously puffy, tired eyes. Not such a great way to say "good morning"! Under-eye puffiness is usually due to fluid accumulation in that area. Sometimes, it's from allergies; other times, heredity; but most often—at least for me—sleep deprivation, dehydration, and/or alcohol consumption are to blame. Whatever the cause, one of the best ways to banish under-eye bags is with this cooling sea salt treatment that absorbs excess fluid and fights inflammation.

Makes 1 treatment

1 teaspoon sea salt
1 cup warm water

1. Combine the sea salt and warm water in a small bowl or jar. Stir or shake until the salt has dissolved.

2. Cut a cotton pad to fit the eye area, soak it in the saltwater solution, then put the cotton pad in the freezer for a few minutes until icy cold.

3. Apply to the eye area, let sit for 15 minutes, then remove. Follow with your favorite eye cream.

SEA SALT ACNE TREATMENT

Have you ever noticed how your skin looks especially great after a day at the beach? And even better after a week? Sure, de-stressing can do wonders to clear up a cranky complexion, but more than likely it's the magic of seawater that's giving you that glow—acne sufferers know what I'm talking about. Salt, as we know, has absorbent properties and is, therefore, really good at clearing out pores, making it especially effective against stubborn blackheads and pimples.

But beyond cleansing, salt is a powerful blemish buster, thanks to its antibacterial and pH-balancing properties. Just think about salted fish or meats—they don't require refrigeration, because bacteria doesn't survive well in a highly salty environment. Even if you don't live near the ocean, you can enjoy the acne-fighting skin benefits of seawater at home with this DIY facial. Himalayan pink salt is my first choice for this treatment, with its more than 84 minerals that will boost your skin health, but any good-quality sea salt will work. Just remember to let the mixture cool before applying it to your skin, because burns + acne = a big mess you don't want to deal with.

Makes about 1 cup acne treatment

1 cup water

3 tablespoons sea salt

1. Bring the water to a boil in a small saucepan. Remove from the heat, add the sea salt, and stir to dissolve.

2. Allow the salt water to cool to room temperature, or until cool enough to comfortably handle.

3. To use: Dip a cotton ball or soft cloth in the mixture and gently rub it over freshly cleaned skin. Allow the salt water to remain on the skin for 15 minutes—it will dry.

4. Rinse thoroughly with warm water, pat dry, and follow with a moisturizer.

MAKEUP REMOVER PADS

You know those days when you're so utterly *done* by bedtime that the idea of brushing your teeth and washing your face feels like a Herculean undertaking? I'm with you—and the piece of bedtime beauty routine that tends to feel most daunting to me in that all-too-frequent state of existence is makeup removal. I've figured out, however, that I can trick myself into taking care of my skin even when I'm exhausted by keeping a handy stash of makeup remover pads at the ready. But rather than shell out for prepackaged, chemical-laden face cleaning wipes, I make my own. With just a few nourishing ingredients, these pads feel great and—most important—work unbelievably well for removing dirt and makeup. Yes, even waterproof mascara. Raccoon eyes and smudged pillowcases begone!

Makes about 2 weeks' worth of pads

1 cup hot water

2 tablespoons extra virgin olive oil

2 tablespoons natural liquid face wash

1 teaspoon witch hazel

5 drops tea tree essential oil

5 drops grapefruit essential oil

1. Combine the water, olive oil, face wash, witch hazel, and essential oils in a small mason jar or other lidded container. Stir or shake well.

2. Add as many round cotton pads to the liquid as you can fit in the jar. They will quickly absorb the liquid in the jar. Cover and store at room temperature for up to 2 weeks.

Note: Tea tree oil is a natural preservative and will extend the shelf life of your pads. If you want to keep them longer than 2 weeks, refrigerate them.

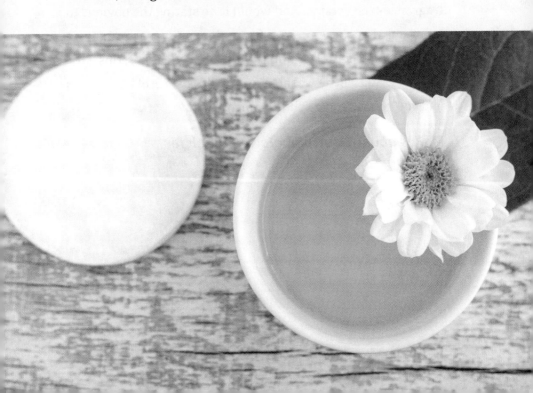

LIP BALM

If there's one product out there that I think is easy enough for *anyone* to make at home, it's lip balm. Yep, even you! This one has a mere four ingredients (5 if you opt to add essential oils) and is really just a simple melt-and-pour undertaking. I'm telling you it will take you all of about 10 minutes to make, including cleanup, and results in about 20 tubes of lip balm (or a few larger pots—you can store this however you like). Made with hydrating olive and coconut oils to leave lips feeling soft and supple, vitamin E—a workhorse of a vitamin—to heal and fight free radicals, and beeswax to create a silky smooth texture, this balm will not only moisturize, but also protect lips against the elements.

You can customize the balm with a few drops of essential oil in whatever scent you like or leave that out entirely for a fragrance-free version. And would it be stating the obvious to point out that these make a fantastic party favor or holiday gift? The internet is brimming with cute little tubes, tins, jars, and pots! Add a little washi tape or tie on a sprig of fresh herbs and you're ready to brighten someone's day.

Makes about 1 cup lip balm—enough for about 20 tubes

¼ cup extra virgin olive oil

¼ cup coconut oil

2 tablespoons beeswax pastilles

½ teaspoon vitamin E oil

5 to 10 drops essential oil of your choice (I like bergamot, rose, or lavender, but use what you like)

1. Place the olive oil, coconut oil, and beeswax in a small, heat-safe bowl or mason jar and place in a small saucepan filled with water. Heat over medium-low heat, stirring, until the mixture is completely melted. Add the vitamin E oil and stir to combine.

2. Remove from the heat and stir in the essential oil(s), then carefully pour into tubes or tins and let set for at least 1 hour.

3. Store in a cool, dry place.

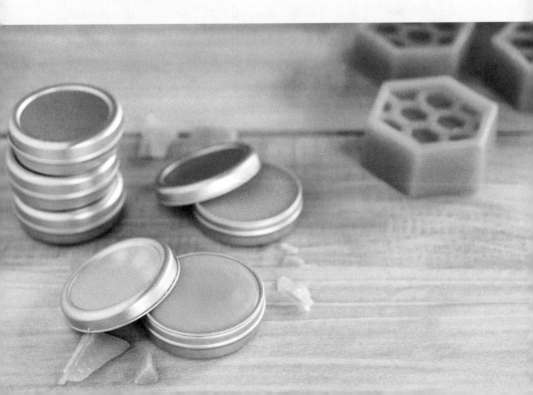

HAND SALVE

I don't know about you, but I wash my hands so often nowadays that I seem to have developed a Pavlovian response to hearing the sound of running water: I automatically start humming the "Happy Birthday" song to myself for 20 seconds. Ah, well, there are worse side effects to having good hand hygiene. I know of one for sure: dry, cracked hands. Yep, as important as it is, all of that hand washing (and hand sanitizing) can really do a number on your skin.

The best and, frankly, only way I know of to combat painfully dry hands is to regularly and religiously use a super rich moisturizer, such as this oil-based salve. It's unbelievably easy to make—literally just a matter of melting some ingredients together—and it moisturizes and protects like crazy, thanks to soothing olive oil and thick, vitamin E–rich shea butter. You can make yours unscented, but adding a few drops of essential oil is a nice touch. Try soothing lavender, cooling eucalyptus, or calming chamomile. For extra moisturizing, slather this salve on at bedtime, pull on a pair of cotton gloves, and wake up to markedly improved hands in the morning.

Makes about 6 ounces salve

3 tablespoons beeswax pastilles or grated beeswax

5 tablespoons shea butter

5 tablespoons olive oil

25 to 30 drops essential oils of your choice (optional)

1. Gently melt the beeswax in a double boiler or a stainless steel bowl set over a pot of simmering water, over medium-low heat. Add the shea butter and allow it to melt completely.

2. Remove the beeswax mixture from the heat and stir in the olive oil and essential oils (if using).

3. Allow the mixture to cool slightly.

4. Pour the salve into a small lidded jar, tin, or other container of your choice and allow it to cool completely.

5. To use: Dip your fingers into the salve and apply it to hands and cuticles. Massage gently until absorbed.

Note: This salve makes a lovely gift. Pour it into pretty little tins, add a decorative label and/or some ribbon, and you're in business!

SCENTED MASSAGE OIL

On gift-giving occasions, some people are just hard to shop for. I like to think I'm not one of those people. I like lots of things! New books, new clothes, new kitchen "toys," tickets to a show. But if ever there were a slam-dunk gift for me, it's a massage. There's little I love more than the total relaxation of that experience. And, of course, beyond the straight-up indulgence of it, there are tons of benefits, including improved circulation, eased muscle tension, and the release of toxins. Add aromatherapy to the picture and a happy, magical kind of synergy takes place. As a result, I've tinkered with making my own massage oil. It's a lovely gift to give and—if you're lucky—just the thing to keep on hand if you happen to live with someone who is willing to offer you a massage at home from time to time. But even in the absence of your own personal on-call masseuse, this oil is great for a quick tension-relieving head and scalp massage (when you've been staring at a screen for too long), foot and calf massage (for those DIY pedicures), or face massage (for keeping that muscle tone!).

Makes about 1 ounce massage oil (about 10 treatments)

¼ cup extra virgin olive oil

20 to 25 drops essential oils (sandalwood, jasmine, and geranium are especially nice, but use what you like)

1. Combine the olive and essential oils in a small lidded jar or bottle. Shake well to mix.

2. To use: Shake well before each use. Pour about 1 teaspoon into your hands and gently massage into skin.

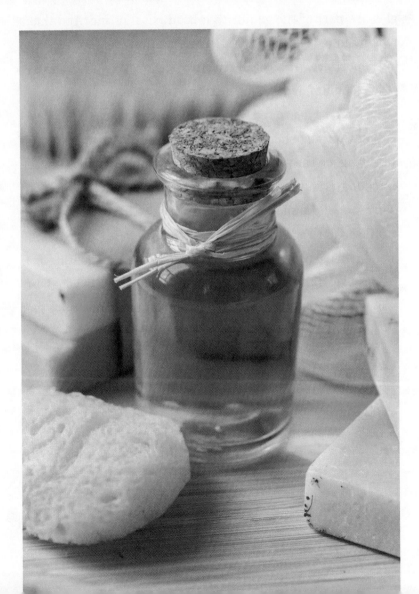

MOISTURIZING BODY WASH

It's no secret that I love a good DIY personal care product—not only for the fun of it, but because it means I can control the ingredients that go into the products I use. Thumb through any of the books I've written and you'll find tons of salves, scrubs, balms, masks, lotions—even homemade makeup! But where I draw the line is at the use of caustic chemicals. If safety goggles are part of the game, it's a hard pass for me. And that's why making soap from scratch has typically not been part of my repertoire. Almost all *real* soap making requires the use of lye (sodium hydroxide), a strong chemical that I'm just too nervous to have around with little kids in the house.

Not wanting to be left out of what seems like such a fun project, I've gone the semihomemade route and stayed within the extended family of soap making, turning out what is essentially souped-up shower gel. Starting with a base of pure liquid castile soap (traditionally made with olive oil), I've combined moisturizing honey, luxe olive oil, and the intoxicating fragrance of vanilla and orange (although you can scent yours any way you want) to create a fabulous foaming shower gel that moisturizes while it cleanses.

Makes about 1 cup body wash

⅓ cup liquid castile soap

⅓ cup raw honey

⅓ cup extra virgin olive oil

15 drops vanilla essential oil (optional)

10 to 15 drops sweet orange essential oil (optional)

1. Combine all the ingredients in a bowl and whisk together until thoroughly mixed.

2. Transfer the mixture to a pump or squeeze-top bottle.

3. Store at room temperature (or in the shower!) for up to 1 year.

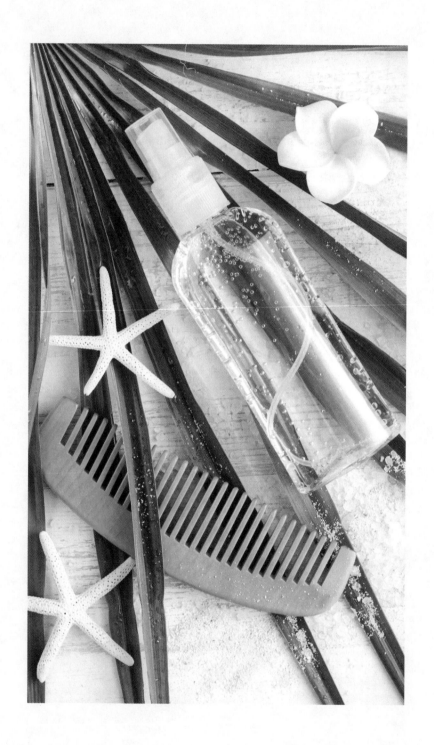

BEACH WAVES SEA SALT HAIRSPRAY

Isn't beach hair the best? Something about the combination of sunshine, salt water, and sticky air is a cocktail for gorgeous, soft waves. And although you can't exactly bottle a perfect day at the beach (oh, if only . . .), re-creating that natural beachy look at home is easier than you might think. This DIY sea salt spray helps create highly texturized locks when there's no surf in sight. Mix it all up together in a spray bottle for the easiest cleanup ever. Start with towel-dried hair, and you're just a handful of ingredients away from those quintessentially seaside locks.

Makes about 1 cup hairspray, enough for quite a few uses

1 cup hot water

2 teaspoons sea salt

1 tablespoon coconut oil

½ teaspoon leave-in conditioner

⅛ teaspoon pomade or styling gel

1. Pour the hot water into a clean spray bottle.

2. Add the remaining ingredients, screw on the spray nozzle, and shake well to combine.

3. To use: Shake well, then spray liberally on towel-dried hair, scrunch, twist (and scrunch some more). Air dry or blow dry.

DEEP-CONDITIONING HAIR MASK

Perhaps you think about hair masks in the same way I think about washing windows: I know it's a good thing to do, I'll be happy when it's done, but it takes too long and I don't have time. I get it. You already wash and condition your hair and doing a mask feels like yet another step in an already complicated beauty routine—so many products, so little time. But here's the thing: this mask is super quick to mix up and delivers results that are more than worth the investment of time (which is all of 15 minutes, by the way). And what's even better is that the ingredient list consists of a mere two items, both of which are likely sitting on your kitchen counter right now: banana and olive oil.

Banana is great for all hair types, but works particularly well on dull, damaged, or dry hair—as it's rich in vitamins and minerals (such as potassium) that can strengthen the hair and balance the pH of the scalp. Olive oil, rich in healthy fats and vitamin E, helps repair damage that causes breakage and split ends and makes the hair look shiny and sleek.

But let's answer the real question, shall we? The one that you're asking yourself right now. *What the heck am I supposed to do for 15 minutes while I wait for this stuff to work?* Here are eight ideas:

Mask your face, too (see page 206 for an easy and effective homemade facial mask).

- Paint your nails.
- Shave your legs.
- Clean the bathroom.
- Catch up on e-mails.
- Meditate, stretch.
- Take a bath.
- Call a friend—like on the actual phone, old school, with your voice.

Makes 1 treatment

1 banana
1 tablespoon olive oil

1. Combine the banana and olive oil in a bowl. Using a fork, mash together until the mixture is smooth and creamy.

2. While in the shower, apply the mask to your hair and scalp with fingers. Leave on for 10 to 15 minutes before rinsing.

HOT OIL TREATMENT FOR HAIR AND SCALP

Lest you think a "hot oil treatment" might involve dumping piping hot oil over your head, rest assured, it's nothing like that. This beauty trick, whereby gently warmed oil is massaged into the hair and scalp, is the *answer* to your hair's 911 call (and not the other way around).

Heat styling, color-treating, sun exposure, wind, and surf can all leave hair dry, brittle, damaged, and desperate for some TLC. Applying warm olive oil to stressed locks helps strengthen, protect, and moisturize them. With regular use (once a week is ideal), your hair will be healthier, your scalp and hair will be less dry, you'll have less frizz and flyaways, and fewer split ends. This is all a huge bonus if you're trying to grow out your hair, because healthy hair = longer hair. Pro tip: Heat the oil in a squeeze bottle set in a bowl of warm water for the easiest application.

Makes 1 treatment

1 tablespoon to ¼ cup extra virgin olive oil, depending
    on hair length

About 1 cup water

1. Place the olive oil in a squeeze bottle (or bowl if you don't
   have one).

2. Place the water in a microwave-safe bowl and microwave
   for 30 to 45 seconds, until steaming but not scalding.

3. Set the squeeze bottle in the hot water until the oil inside
   is warm to the touch—test a few drops on your wrist first
   to make sure it's a comfortable temperature.

4. To use: Section your hair and apply the treatment generously to damp or dry hair from roots to ends. Massage the
   product into your scalp. Cover your hair with a shower
   cap and/or a warm towel. Leave the oil in for 30 minutes
   before washing your hair with shampoo and conditioner.

CUTICLE OIL

A gorgeous manicure isn't just about the polish; great-looking nails mean soft and supple cuticles, too. Because we all know that even when you do manage to find the perfect shade, having dry, cracked, or jagged cuticles can totally ruin an otherwise marvelous mani.

When your nails are in need of a little TLC and you can't get to the salon right away—or when you *have* been to the nail salon and want to keep your manicure looking fresh—this DIY treatment, with nourishing olive oil and antibacterial tea tree oil, is just the thing to keep your cuticles in tip-top shape and to prevent your polish from cracking. This treatment is especially easy to use with one of those handy little roller bottles. They're inexpensive and readily available online. You see? Now you've (ahem) nailed it!

Makes several treatments

8 drops tea tree essential oil
2 teaspoons extra virgin olive oil

1. Place the tea tree oil in a 10 ml roller bottle, roller ball removed, then fill the bottle the rest of the way with the olive oil. Shake well to mix.

2. To use: Apply a small amount of cuticle oil to each fingertip once a day, rubbing it into your cuticles and fingernails. Use daily.

BEARD OIL

If you think olive oil works well to tame the hair on your head, you should see what it can do for facial hair! No, it's not a ton of work to maintain a beard, but there *is* some upkeep: regular washing, trimming, and moisturizing. As beard hair is typically pretty coarse, men often experience itchiness, dry skin, and even ingrown hairs on the skin underneath. Not only that, long beards can become quite tangled and unruly and, therefore, need to be combed to keep them looking good.

Beard oil goes a long way to make smoothing, detangling, and taming facial hair an easier task, not to mention what it offers the skin hiding underneath. A simple mixture of olive oil, jojoba oil, and a few well-chosen essential oils is all it takes to soften and tame beard scruff while leaving behind a faint masculine scent. Make it yourself, like this:

Makes about 3 tablespoons beard oil

2 tablespoons olive oil

1 tablespoon jojoba oil (avocado, grapeseed, or argan oil work well, too)

15 to 30 drops of essential oil, such as bay, cedarwood, lemongrass, or fir

1. Combine all the ingredients in a small lidded bowl or jar. Shake well to mix. Store in a cool, dark place.

2. To use: Simply pour a few drops into your hand and rub it into a freshly washed beard, then comb, if desired.

HOUSEHOLD
USES

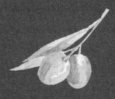

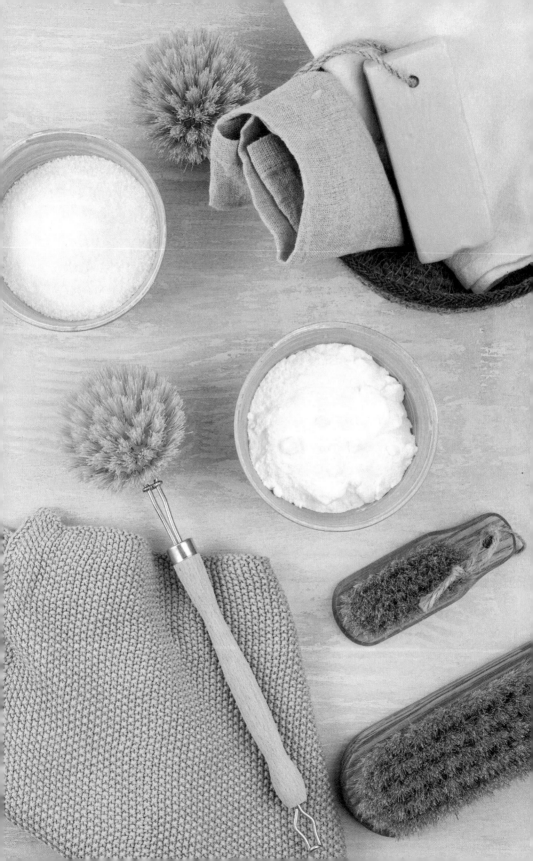

PRODUCE WASH

We all know how important it is to wash our hands and kitchen surfaces after touching poultry or meat, to avoid cross-contamination and food-borne illnesses (a.k.a. food poisoning), but did you know that washing produce is just as important? According to the FDA, about 48 million people get sick from contaminated food each year. Eek! That's 1 in 6 people! And it's not all from eating contaminated meat. Fresh produce can carry bacteria, too. To keep your family safe and healthy, follow these simple tips, including washing all fruits and vegetables in salt water, to ensure they're as clean as possible before you eat them.

Makes 1 treatment

About 1 teaspoon sea salt for every cup of water used

1. Wash your hands for 20 seconds with warm water and soap before and after handling fresh produce.

2. Fill a very clean sink or large bowl with clean, cool water. Add about 1 teaspoon of sea salt for every cup of water—you can eyeball this. Stir to combine.

3. Add fresh produce to the saltwater bath and let it sit for 10 to 15 minutes, then rinse with cool water.

4. Dry produce with *clean* kitchen towels or paper towels.

5. Store cut produce, berries, greens, or other delicate fruits and vegetables at 40°F or below.

QUICK-CHILLER FOR WINE OR CHAMPAGNE

If I had a dollar for every time I've forgotten to chill a bottle of white wine before dinner guests arrived, I'd be rich. Rich and drunk on warm wine. Well, maybe just the warm wine part. If you can relate, I have great news. Plunging a bottle of wine into a bucket of salted ice water chills it in mere minutes. Adding salt lowers the water's freezing point, which makes the cooling process super efficient. So, the next time you forget to cool that bottle of white, rose, or bubbly, this trick will help you—and your wine—chill out in no time.

Chills 1 bottle

1 cup sea salt
Ice

1. Set your bottle of wine in an ice bucket or large metal bowl (the bowl of a stand mixer works well in a pinch) and fill with ice.

2. Pour cold water over the ice.

3. Add the salt and gently stir to incorporate.

4. Twist the bottle in the ice bath every few minutes and you should find that the wine is chilled in under 10 minutes. Cheers!

WOODEN CUTTING BOARD CLEANER

As you might expect of a cookbook author, I own a bunch of cutting boards in a variety of sizes and material. My most prized, however, is a huge, wooden butcher block board that remains permanently stationed on my countertop. It is my favorite for several reasons. I like its durability and the fact that it is actually *less* likely to harbor bacteria than the plastic ones (true fact! See my book *The Baking Soda Companion* for more on that). I like its impressive heft and—more than anything—I just love the way it looks. To keep it clean, I give it a daily wipe with a little soap and water or vinegar, but to keep it stain-free and smelling fresh, I give it a good cleaning every couple of days with salt and lemon juice. The salt is a great natural abrasive and the acid in the lemon juice helps keep odor-causing bacteria at bay. Plus it smells good!

Makes 1 treatment

A small handful of coarse sea salt

½ lemon

1. Spread a handful of coarse salt on a dry wooden cutting board.

2. Holding the lemon half cut side down, use it to scrub the salt over the surface of the wood, gently squeezing the lemon to release its juice as you go.

3. Once you've thoroughly scrubbed the board, let the juice and salt sit for 5 minutes. Rinse off the board in the sink with running water or use a wet sponge to clean off any residue.

4. Allow the cutting board to air dry.

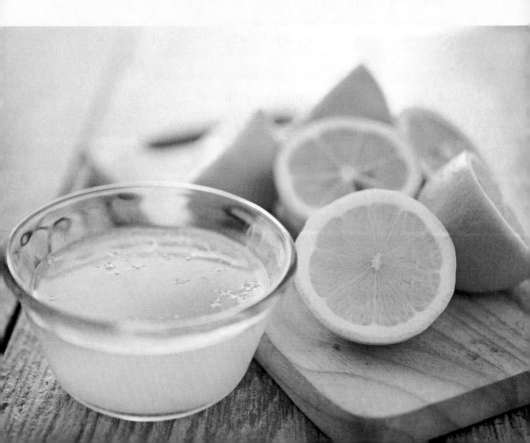

WINE STAIN REMOVER

It happens. You've got guests for dinner. The conversation is flowing, and so is the wine. The next thing you know, someone (no, of course not *you*) has spilled red wine on your couch, your rug, or (gasp!) your dress. Don't panic! First, take a breath. No, not another sip—a breath! And move fast, because red wine will sink and settle into those fibers the longer it's there. Also, you're going to need to resist the urge to rub like crazy. This is where not panicking is a good idea. Take another breath. Okay, go ahead, take a sip if that helps. Now, follow these simple instructions for diluting and wicking that wine right off the fabric with the help of sea salt, and then get back to your party!

Makes 1 treatment

Sea salt—amount varies, depending on the size of stain
Boiling water

1. Blot the stain to remove excess liquid.

2. Pour sea salt over the stain and allow it to settle for several minutes.

3. Pour boiling water over the stain and blot again.

KITCHEN SPONGE REVIVER

Doing dishes is a dirty job—even dirtier if the sponge you use hasn't been cleaned in a while! Kitchen sponges can be a hotbed for bacteria. No surprise there; sponges are moist and full of dirt and food particles. What better breeding ground for bacteria? So it's important to clean them—or replace them—on a regular basis.

A good rule of thumb is this: When a sponge starts to stink, it's time to say goodbye. You can, however, extend the time it takes to get to that point of disgustingness by giving it a regular soak in salt water. Salt, through osmosis, sucks the water out of many types of bacteria, effectively killing it. And when it comes to sponges, the best way to get the salt deep into all those dark and nasty crevices is by soaking them in a salty solution, like so.

Makes 1 treatment

¼ cup sea salt
1 quart water

1. Combine the salt and water in a medium bowl or other container. Stir until the salt dissolves. Submerge the sponge and allow it to soak overnight.

2. The next morning, wring out as much water as possible and allow the sponge to dry.

STAINLESS STEEL CLEANER

Do you have stainless steel appliances in your kitchen? Oh, you do? Then you probably have *smudged* stainless steel appliances in your kitchen, as I do. Stainless is a great surface for kitchen appliances in many ways. Sure, it's durable and attractive, but actually stainless? I beg to differ. The good news is that there's a ridiculously easy way to get rid of those fingerprints, streaks, and water stains. And it's olive oil for the win! Just a few drops is all it takes to leave your stainless steel shiny, sparkling, and streak-free. But do me a favor, will you? Please don't use your top-shelf finishing oil here. This is definitely a job for a less expensive workhorse of an oil.

Makes 1 treatment

A few drops of olive oil

1. Place a few drops of olive oil on a clean, soft cloth (microfiber is ideal).

2. Use the cloth to gently buff your stainless steel, working in the same direction as the grain (look closely to see in which direction it runs). Rub until smudges and other marks are gone.

3. Finish by rubbing the metal with a clean, dry cloth.

CAST-IRON SKILLET CLEANER

Few tools in my kitchen are as prized or as beloved as my cast-iron skillet. It's durable, distributes heat like a dream, works equally well on the stovetop and in the oven, and, although it sounds a little crazy to say so, it is the only piece of cookware I own that has a personality. I love her (yes, *her*!) and, as such, make sure to take special care of her. My regular maintenance is a very simple two-part process. I clean her with salt and season her with olive oil. And I never—never ever *ever*—wash her with soap. It's the cardinal sin of cast iron maintenance. If you have a cast-iron skillet, please, *step away from the soap*. That aside, with proper care, a cast-iron skillet can last nearly forever, and really only gets better with age. To keep yours in tip-top shape, follow these easy steps.

Makes 1 treatment

1 cup coarse sea salt
About 1 tablespoon olive oil

1. Pour the coarse salt into the still-warm skillet. Using a kitchen towel or paper towel, scour the pan until all stuck-on food is removed.

2. Discard the salt and rinse the skillet with warm water.

3. Dry the pan immediately.

4. Using a cloth or paper towel, rub a light coat of olive oil on the inside of the skillet. Buff to remove any excess.

COPPER CLEANER

Copper is considered by many to be the (*ahem*) gold standard when it comes to cookware. It is often touted as the best material in which to whisk egg whites for meringue, thanks to a special reaction that takes place between the metal and the egg whites. Its quick response to temperature change makes it a dream for sautéing and even more so for heating sugar for caramel or candy making, which requires a great deal of precision. Given that, you'd think everyone's kitchen would be brimming with copper cookware. And it would, except for one little hitch—it's expensive. So, if you do make the investment in copper—or are lucky enough to inherit some—you'll want to put in the time to maintain it. And that's the other thing about copper. It will tarnish. Guaranteed. Thankfully, it's easy to polish away with just two nontoxic household items: salt and lemons. This method works almost instantly, restoring copper's gleaming beauty in the blink of an eye.

Makes 1 treatment

3 tablespoons fresh lemon juice

1 tablespoon fine sea salt

1. Combine the lemon juice and fine salt in a small bowl. Stir until the salt dissolves.

2. Dip a soft cloth into the mixture and wipe the copper.

3. Continue to rub the surface and apply more of the salt solution as needed until tarnish is removed.

4. Rinse the copper clean with warm water. Dry thoroughly.

5. Buff with a dry, clean cloth, if desired.

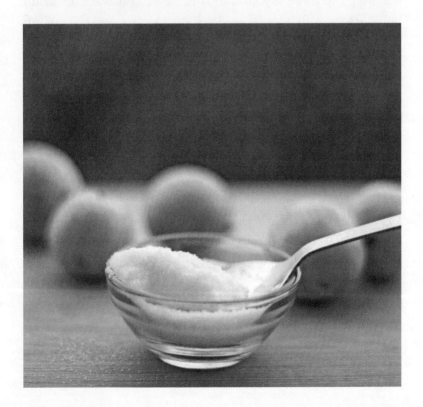

DRAIN DECLOGGER

My husband and I are the fortunate parents of two lovely girls. We worry about them, of course, as parents do, although not necessarily about the same things. My husband started worrying about our future shower drain problems when our girls were both still in diapers and he realized that 75 percent of our household might someday have long hair. I teased him at the time, but it turns out he was right. We have drain issues. This summer, as we once again found ourselves standing in water up to our ankles in the shower and weren't able to get a plumber to come, my husband decided to excavate the drain himself and pulled out something the likes of which . . . oh, I'll spare you the details.

We determined then and there that regularly and preemptively treating our drains was the way to go, but we wanted to do so without commercial drain cleaners—they're full of sodium hydroxide or sulfuric acid, which are harsh and could eat away at our pipes over time, not to mention the ickiness of exposing ourselves to those chemicals. Instead, we've turned to a powerful yet nontoxic cocktail of salt, baking soda, and vinegar that blasts through hair and gunk to get the water flowing properly again. No haircuts required!

Makes 1 treatment

1 cup baking soda

1 cup sea salt

1 cup white vinegar

1. Pour the baking soda down the drain, followed by the sea salt and the vinegar. (Watch out! It will foam.)

2. Allow the mixture to sit for 10 to 15 minutes, then flush it with a pot of boiling water.

3. At this point, the drain should be clear! If not, repeat the process until water drains freely.

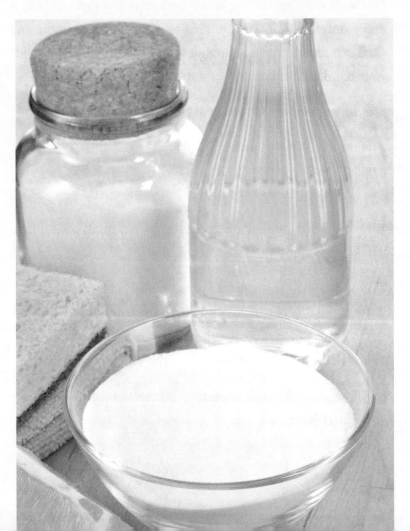

DIY WALL SPACKLE

Anyone who has lived in as many different apartments as I did, once upon a time, knows a thing or two about filling nail holes at the last minute on move-out day. From toothpaste to school glue, I've tried a lot of DIY spackle in the name of getting a full refund on my security deposit. But the one I found to work best is a miraculous paste made from salt and cornstarch. It works on nail holes, chips, and dings on sheetrock or plaster and it dries in about an hour. For a perfectly smooth, good-as-new wall, the spackle can be sanded with 100-grit sandpaper and painted over, once dry. That is, if you have the time and don't, you know, have a moving truck double parked outside your building . . .

Makes enough to fill several holes

2 tablespoons fine sea salt

2 tablespoons cornstarch

1 to 1½ tablespoons water

1. Combine the fine salt and cornstarch in a small bowl with enough water to make a thick paste.

2. Using a putty knife (or any blunt knife—a plastic knife from the takeout restaurant down the block works!), scoop out a tiny amount of spackle and gently push it into the hole. Then, use the flat surface of the knife to smooth it out.

3. Allow the spackle to dry for at least an hour, then sand and paint, if desired.

WOODEN TABLE WATER MARK REMOVER

White rings on wood furniture: sometimes the unfortunate aftermath of good times and a forgotten coaster, sometimes the unfortunate aftermath of takeout wonton soup and the same forgotten coaster. Whether from a sweating cocktail glass or a too-warm mug, these rings happen as a result of moisture soaking into the top layers of the wood finish, then getting trapped beneath the wax and clouding up. They may be an eyesore, but luckily they're usually temporary. One of the quickest, easiest ways to banish water marks on wood is with a simple paste made from salt and water. And when you're finished removing the stain, use a few drops of olive oil on a soft cloth to restore the luster of the wood. And all is well in the world again.

Makes 1 treatment

1 teaspoon fine sea salt
A few drops of water

1. Mix the fine salt with a few drops of water to form a paste.

2. Gently rub the paste onto the water mark with a soft cloth or sponge, working in a circular motion, until the spot is gone.

SLATE, TILE, AND HARDWOOD FLOOR POLISH

Coating a floor in olive oil sounds more like the setup for a prank than a cleaning hack, but I promise this homemade floor polish will leave you with beautiful gleaming floors, not pratfalls. Unlike commercial cleaners, which are full of harsh chemicals that can strip wood or discolor slate and tile, this stuff—made with just lemon juice and olive oil—gently and naturally gets floors looking like new again. Just give your floors a thorough sweep and then follow with a dry mop dipped in just a little bit of the following solution—any remaining dust will cling to the mop like magic. I like to use an old floor sweeper and tuck a microfiber cloth into the indentations that are meant to hold the pad refills in place (the ones I stopped buying ages ago). After that, grab your sunglasses because your floors are gonna shine!

Makes 1 or 2 treatments, depending on the size of the floors

1 tablespoon fresh lemon juice

½ teaspoon olive oil

1. Combine the lemon juice and olive oil in a small bowl. Stir well.

2. Sweep the floor to remove large particles of dirt and dust.

3. Apply about a teaspoon of the olive oil solution to the mop and mop the floor, adding more solution to the mop as needed. Don't pour the solution directly on the floor.

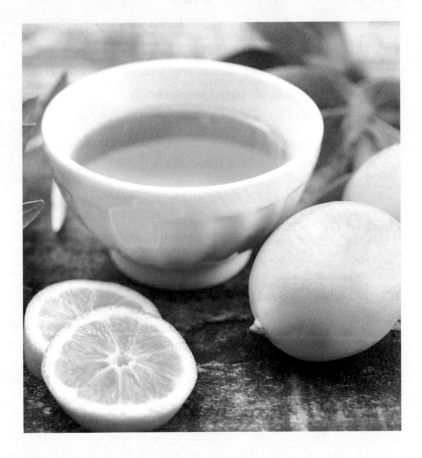

SQUEAKY HINGE LUBRICANT

WD-40 is one of those products that seems like a must-have in every "grown-up" home. It's magical, lubricating stuff and, until recently, I thought it could fix just about anything that was stuck, squeaking, or otherwise nonbudging around the house. We live in a very old home—built in 1905—and, as such, there's a lot of squeaking and creaking around here. Part of the charm? Maybe. What's not charming, however, is a shrieking door hinge, which is what we were dealing with in our bedroom. To fix it, I grabbed for the WD-40, only to find that the can was empty!

So, I decided to consult the internet, as one does in such a pinch, and found that oil-based lubricants (such as petroleum jelly and, well, WD-40) were recommended. Oil-based, hmm . . . I bet you can guess where I went next. You got it: I grabbed a bottle of olive oil, and darn it if I don't have a new favorite way to quiet a squeaky door.

Makes 1 treatment

Olive oil

1. To lubricate a squeaky hinge, drip a small amount of olive oil at the top of the hinge and help the drops of oil run down by moving the hinge back and forth.

2. Keep a clean cloth or rag handy to catch spills and to wipe off the excess.

WOOD FURNITURE CLEANER

There's a small window of time, really just a handful of years, during which kids weirdly think that cleaning is fun. For example, if you hand a kid anywhere between age 4 and 9 a spray bottle and a rag, they will be giddy with excitement. My kids literally fight over who *gets* to clean the coffee table. I'd like to think it's because they love using this homemade furniture polish so much, but deep in my heart I know that it's because the novelty of sprays and suds and brooms and mops has yet to wear off. May it endure forever. Meanwhile, this homemade wood furniture polish (which I'm happy to hand over, because there are no weird chemicals in it) is super effective and takes seconds to make.

Disinfecting white vinegar, conditioning olive oil, and fresh-smelling lemon clean, shine, and protect wood from mild dents and scratches. From chairs and tables to banisters and wooden storage boxes, you can use it on pretty much any wooden surface. But you'll have to fight my kids for the coffee table.

Makes about ¾ cup wood cleaner

½ cup white vinegar

¼ cup olive oil

1 tablespoon fresh lemon juice

20 to 30 drops lavender essential oil (optional, but a nice touch)

1. Combine all the ingredients in a spray bottle. Shake well.

2. Spray on wood and rub with microfiber or other soft cloth.

WICKER FURNITURE PROTECTOR

Lightweight, durable, and super eco-friendly, wicker and rattan furniture makes a stylish statement both indoors and out—that is, until it starts to age. Over time, wicker dries out and starts to look less than stunning. To keep yours looking its best and to help it last, a little maintenance and routine cleaning is all you need. Most of the time, a quick wipe with a mild soap solution is all that's necessary. If your furniture has a lot of dirt and debris, vacuum it with the dust-brush attachment or gently brush it with a clean, dry paintbrush or an old toothbrush. And because sunlight is wicker's archrival, always cover yours if you plan to leave it outside for more than a few weeks at a time. Beyond those steps, one of the best things you can do to keep your wicker looking vibrant is to give it an occasional rubdown with olive oil every six months or so. Just be sure to let it dry well before sitting on wicker chairs—the seat of your pants will thank you.

Makes 1 treatment

Olive oil (amount depends on size and number of pieces of furniture)

1. Dip a clean, soft cloth in olive oil and thoroughly wipe down your wicker furniture.

2. Finish by rubbing the wicker with a clean, dry cloth.

3. Repeat every 6 months.

FLOWER VASE CLEANER

I love fresh flowers and am lucky enough to have a very sweet husband who shows up with pretty blooms on a fairly regular basis for no particular reason. And what do I do to thank him for his thoughtfulness? I leave those cut flowers in their vase just long enough for the water to turn foul, for the petals to start falling off, and for the inside of the vase to become coated with a stinking sludge. Good times. Even after I've disposed of the gross water, the residue left inside the vase can be hard to scrub. Thankfully, a simple paste made from salt and vinegar and a brush is all it takes to get even the narrowest, hardest-to-clean vases sparkling again.

Makes 1 treatment

1½ teaspoons fine sea salt
White vinegar

1. Combine the salt with just enough vinegar to make a paste. Rub it onto the inside of the vase using a sponge, bottle brush, or old toothbrush.

2. Let the mixture sit for 10 minutes before rising the vase with warm water.

3. Dry with a soft towel or microfiber cloth.

ARTIFICIAL PLANT CLEANER

Maybe you don't have a green thumb, or you travel a lot for work. Maybe you have a commitment-phobia or live underground in a windowless Cold War–era bunker that you got for a steal. There are lots of reasons that taking care of live plants may not be for you and, therefore, decorating with artificial greenery makes a lot of sense. Fake plants come with many benefits. For one thing, they're super low maintenance; they don't need water or fertilizer. And their leaves are always green. That said, they do still require some care to keep them looking their best.

Artificial plants collect dust and other gunk much more so than live plants, so they need to be cleaned regularly. For artificial houseplants, follow these easy steps using olive oil to enhance their shine and to keep them looking like the real McCoy. And for silk flowers, use the handy dry-clean approach to remove dust from hard to reach places with salt. Then sit back, relax, and enjoy the serenity that a touch of nature brings to your bunker.

Makes 1 treatment

FOR SILK FLOWERS

½ cup coarse sea salt

FOR PLASTIC PLANTS

Several drops of olive oil

To clean silk flowers:

1. Pour the sea salt into a resealable plastic bag large enough to accommodate your floral arrangement.

2. Place the silk flowers inside the bag and seal it.

3. Shake the bag vigorously for 1 to 2 minutes.

4. Open the bag, shake the flowers to remove the salt, and return them to their container.

To clean plastic plants:

1. Put a couple of drops of olive oil on a soft cloth or paper towel.

2. Use the cloth to gently polish the plastic.

3. Wipe away the excess oil with a clean cloth.

COSTUME JEWELRY CLEANER

Years ago, when Prince William was to marry Kate Middleton, a very kitschy commercial selling a "genuine replica" of her famous sapphire and diamond engagement ring (the one originally worn by William's mother, Princess Diana) began to air *constantly* on TV. The ring, made with "simulated sapphire" and "scintillating X-4 cubic zirconium" was sold for a whopping $19.90—or, as the exaggerated British voiceover told us, "nineteen dollars ninety."

My husband and I found the whole thing endlessly entertaining so, naturally, when our anniversary came around that year—an occasion for which we'd set a $20 spending limit—my gift pretty much bought itself. That's right, I am now the proud owner of *The Royal Heirloom Ring*. Don't believe me? Check out my Certificate of Authenticity. I joke, but I have to admit I've worn that seen-on-TV ring more often than you might think. It's actually a fun piece of costume jewelry! And while I do keep it safe and sound in its "hinged decorative velveteen jeweler's box," I've found that it needs a bit of TLC every now and again to keep it sparkling. To care for your finest fake bling, use this cleaning method that's gentle enough to remove tarnish and to restore the luster of simulated gemstones without stripping that "authentic" faux finish.

Makes enough to clean several pieces of jewelry

¼ teaspoon baby shampoo or another mild liquid cleanser

¼ cup lukewarm water

1 teaspoon olive oil

½ teaspoon fresh lemon juice

1. Combine the baby shampoo and lukewarm water in a small bowl. Dip a soft toothbrush or cotton swab in the solution and gently rub away dirt and grime from jewelry. Thoroughly dry each piece by patting gently with paper towels.

2. In a separate container, combine the olive oil and lemon juice. Dip a soft cloth or paper towel, wring it out so that it doesn't drip, and gently polish the jewelry. Rinse, then dry.

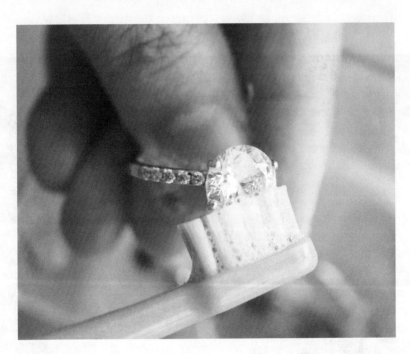

WINDSHIELD DEICER

Anyone who lives in a part of the country where the weather gets cold in the winter knows the annoyance that comes with warming up your car in the morning. I will confess that I am spoiled by my husband, who quite often deices my windows and warms up the car for me when it's especially frigid out so I don't have to stand outside in the freezing air, eyes tearing, cursing the weather. To thank him for this and to make his life a bit easier, I make sure we always have a bottle of this sea salt deicer spray at the ready (aren't I a romantic gift-giver?). Not only does it make quick work of cleaning off the windshield (salt water freezes at lower temperatures than fresh water,

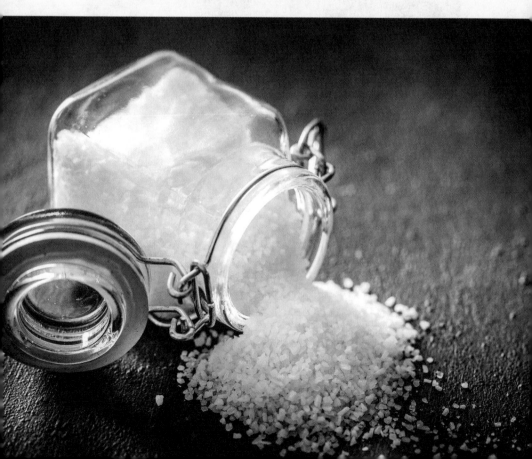

melting the ice right away), it won't cause scratches and other damages that window scrapers can bring about. With a brush, the windshield wipers, and this spray, even the coldest mornings are a little easier to handle.

Makes about 2 cups deicer

2 cups water
2 tablespoons sea salt

1. Combine the water and sea salt in a spray bottle. Shake until the salt is dissolved.

2. To use: Spray the solution on your windshield, being careful to keep the salt on the glass and not on any metal parts, as salt can be corrosive over time. Once the frost and/or ice has melted, turn on your windshield wipers to clear the glass.

IRON RESIDUE REMOVER

I think we can all agree that ironing doesn't top the list of Most Fun Pastimes. And if that's the case, then cleaning an iron ... um ... well, actually, cleaning an iron is kind of surprisingly satisfying. No matter how you feel about ironing, the fact is that if you iron often, the bottom of your iron is eventually going to show its age, and it's best to clean it before iron marks start to show up and ruin your clothes.

Believe it or not, cleaning an iron (without burning your fingers!) is totally possible and requires little more than some sea salt. It will remove stains and dislodge any melted-on fibers left behind by previous jobs so they won't transfer to your clothes. It's a quick fix that'll get you back to that really fun ironing party in no time.

Makes 1 treatment

Brown paper bag or sheet of parchment paper
1 to 2 tablespoons coarse sea salt

1. Set your iron to the hottest setting and lay out a paper bag or piece of parchment on your ironing board.

2. Sprinkle 1 tablespoon of the coarse salt over the paper and iron in a circular motion for about a minute.

3. Repeat, as necessary, with more salt, until the metal plate is clean.

BASEBALL MITT CONDITIONER

This year, we bought our daughter her first baseball mitt. It was a big milestone, especially for my husband, who had waited a long time to play catch in the backyard. The new mitt is purple—her favorite color—and really suits her perfectly. His, on the other hand? Let's just say that the most action it's seen in the last 20 years is as the 15th guy on a 15-person team in a mostly middle-aged dads community softball league. With a lot of wear and tear—some cracking, some stiffening of the leather—it had seen better days, so I decided to bring it back to life. First, I gave it a good cleaning with some store-bought saddle soap (easy to use and to find at hardware stores, drugstores, and online), then a moisturizing and conditioning rubdown with olive oil, as described here. Good as new! His name may not creep up that roster, but at least it won't be his glove's fault.

Makes 1 treatment

Olive oil

1. Apply a few drops of olive oil to a soft cloth—never directly to the leather—and work it into the dry areas of the leather.

2. Let it set for roughly 30 minutes, then wipe away any excess.

3. Play ball!

SHOE POLISH

I have vivid childhood memories of watching my dad polish his shoes. I remember the brush he used, the cloth, and the little tins of shoe polish he kept in a box in his closet. I remember listening to him talk about how carefully he'd shine his boots when he was in the army and the stories he told about growing up in a family that owned a shoe store. He spent decades wearing a suit and tie to work every day and his dress shoes were always well cared for, thanks to the ritual that had become so well embedded into his life. I wonder, do many people still polish their shoes? In a world so full of flip flops and sneakers, shoe shining doesn't seem to be nearly as ubiquitous as it once was.

In my house, shoe shining is certainly a rare thing, even though I love that sort of ritual and tradition. So, driven by equal parts nostalgia and practicality, I do give some of our dress shoes a spiff up every now and again, although I'll confess that I don't keep shoe polish on hand for that purpose. Instead, I use a bit of olive oil to naturally clean and shine them. As it turns out, it's a really effective way to maintain your shoes.

Makes 1 treatment

Olive oil

1. Use a clean, damp rag to clean off any dust from the shoe.

2. Apply a few small drops of olive oil to a soft cloth and buff the shoe to bring out the shine.

PAINT AND MARKER REMOVER FOR SKIN

When my daughter was not quite 3, she woke up one day and decided that she wanted her then-green bedroom walls to be pink, her favorite color. And in typical 3-year-old fashion, she wanted them that way *now*. She refused to play in her room, she refused to nap in her room, and she absolutely would not even consider sleeping in her room until it was pink. But boy, I needed that kid to nap! So, we bee-lined for the hardware store, picked out the most saccharine shade of cotton candy pink in stock, and popped that paint can open ASAP. She and her sister had a slumber party that night while my husband and I painted her room until almost midnight.

Too exhausted to shower, I fell into bed covered in blotches and drops of Pepto-Bismol pink, knowing full well that it would take more than a bar of soap to get my skin clean in the morning. I tried nail polish remover and rubbing alcohol—neither worked. But what *did* work? Olive oil! And it turns out it works on permanent marker, too! Just follow up with hand soap to remove the greasiness and you're back in business.

Makes 1 treatment

Olive oil

Rub a bit of olive oil into the affected skin, wait a minute or two, then wash the skin with soap and water.

STICKER GUNK REMOVER

I have a bit of an obsession with saving jars. Pickle jars, jam jars, honey jars, peanut butter jars. I have a hard time parting with them once I've come to the end of what was originally in them, so I tend to clean and reuse them regularly. But the most annoying bit of this process is the adhesive residue left over from jar labels, price tags, product labels, and (inevitably in my house) kid's stickers. That stuff clings to glassware, toys, and electronics. What a pain! If, like me, you're constantly trying to remove that gluey gunk from jars and other surfaces around your house, resist the urge to go after it with a knife or other scraping tool, which could damage the surface of whatever you're trying to clean. Instead, reach for your bottle of olive oil and remove the goo from glass, plastic, wood, or metal, like so.

Makes 1 treatment

1 to 2 teaspoons olive oil

1. Apply about a teaspoon of olive oil to a paper towel and lay it over the adhesive residue that you'd like to remove.

2. Leave it for several minutes, allowing the oil to dissolve the stubborn glue. Remove the paper towel and rub sticker residue with a clean, dry paper towel or a plastic scraper.

3. Wash away the olive oil with mild soap and water.

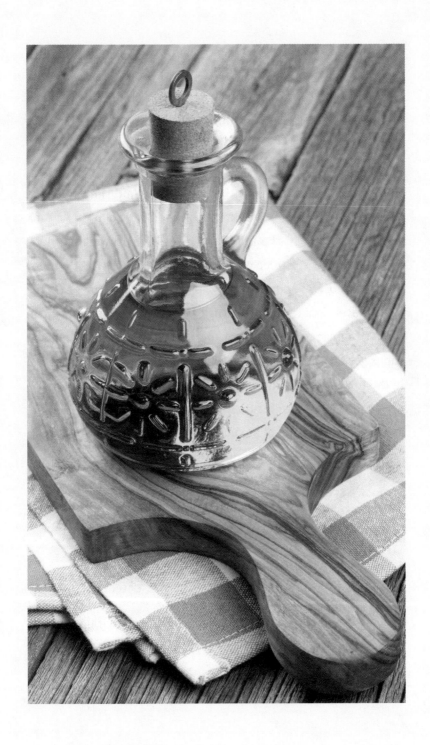

STUCK ZIPPER REMEDY

I have to admit that zippers are one of those staples of everyday life that I have often taken for granted. This, despite the fact that they are absolutely everywhere—from jeans and jackets to suitcases and lunch boxes. They make our lives easier on a daily basis. That is, until they get stuck. And then they are the most frustrating contraptions on the whole planet! A stuck lunch box zipper in the middle of morning rush-out-the-door time? *Arrgh!* The zipper on your dress that just won't budge? *Get me out of this thing!* A boot zipper that won't close? *Oh my gosh!* More often than not, a stuck zipper happens when a little piece of fabric gets caught in the zipper's teeth and then the slider gets stuck. To get it unstuck, you need a bit of lubrication in the form of something slippery, like . . . yes, olive oil! So, the next time you're late for an important meeting and find yourself on the losing end of a stuck zipper situation, let that trusty bottle of olive oil come to your rescue.

Makes 1 treatment

Olive oil

1. Place a few drops of olive oil inside the zipper slider (the "pully" thing that joins the two sets of teeth).

2. Wiggle and work the slider up and down until it becomes "unstuck."

3. Wipe away any excess oil.

CREDITS

Page 12: © SarapulSar38/iStockPhoto.com

Page 16: © apomares/iStockPhoto.com

Page 18 and 183: © dulezidar/iStockPhoto.com

Page 21: © Milan Krasula/iStockPhoto.com

Page 28: © Svetlana_Angelus/iStockPhoto.com

Page 36: © YelenaYemchuk/iStockPhoto.com

Page 38: © jirkaejc/iStockPhoto.com

Page 41, 115, and 256: © fcafotodigital/iStockPhoto.com

Page 45: © Kateryna Ovcharenko/iStockPhoto.com

Page 49: © 5PH/iStockPhoto.com

Page 50 and 213: © kazmulka/iStockPhoto.com

Page 55: © Tatyana Grigoryan/iStockPhoto.com

Page 58 and 67: © Fascinadora/iStockPhoto.com

Page 61: © Lena_Zajchikova/iStockPhoto.com

Page 63: © Nungning20/iStockPhoto.com

Page 72: © AnastasiaNurullina/iStockPhoto.com

Page 78: © LOVE_LIFE/iStockPhoto.com

Page 83: © billnoll/iStockPhoto.com

Page 87: © Mariha-kitchen/iStockPhoto.com

Page 92: © Bartosz Luczak/iStockPhoto.com

Page 97: © Lisovskaya/iStockPhoto.com

Page 109: © OlgaMiltsova/iStockPhoto.com

Page 111: © margouillatphotos/iStockPhoto.com

Page 122: © etorres69/iStockPhoto.com

Page 127 and 136: © bhofack2/iStockPhoto.com

Page 133: © Roxiller/iStockPhoto.com

Page 143: © -lvinst-/iStockPhoto.com

Page 150: © Aamulya/iStockPhoto.com

Page 158: © sbossert/iStockPhoto.com

Page 165: © CarlaMc/iStockPhoto.com

Page 168: © AnthiaCumming/iStockPhoto.com

Page 173: © mythja/iStockPhoto.com

Page 176: © icarmen13/iStockPhoto.com

Page 181: © Andrea Migliarini/iStockPhoto.com

Page 186: © Photopips/iStockPhoto.com

Page 191 and 247: © GSPictures/iStockPhoto.com

Page 197: © Helin Loik-Tomson/iStockPhoto.com

Page 201: © Alikaj2582/iStockPhoto.com

Page 205: © EasterBunnyUK/iStockPhoto.com

Page 207: © Cat_Chat/iStockPhoto.com

Page 215: © Premyuda Yospim/iStockPhoto.com

Page 219: © VieCreative/iStockPhoto.com

Page 222: © Anna-Ok/iStockPhoto.com

Page 231: © netrun78/iStockPhoto.com

Page 235: © rez-art/iStockPhoto.com

Page 241: © undefined undefined/iStockPhoto.com

Page 243: © Geo-grafika/iStockPhoto.com

Page 255: © Kwangmoozaa/iStockPhoto.com

Page 263: © karandaev/iStockPhoto.com

INDEX

*Page numbers in *italics* indicated photographs.

FLAVOR AND SAVOR YOUR FOOD, SUPPORT YOUR HEALTH, AND CLEAN YOUR HOUSE WITH OLIVE OIL AND SEA SALT.

Olive oil and sea salt are common pantry staples, and their versatility knows no bounds. Not only do they make our favorite foods taste great but they have also been used for centuries to supply necessary minerals and boost heart and brain health. Here are 100 recipes for delicious meals and home remedies for healing, beauty, and cleaning, such as:

Kimchi	Sunburn Soother
Salt and Pepper Shrimp	Beach Waves Sea Salt Spray
Olive Oil Chocolate Mousse	Wine Stain Remover

The Olive Oil & Sea Salt Companion is your one-stop shop for delicious, easy, and fun recipes for everyday routines.

ALSO BY SUZY SCHERR

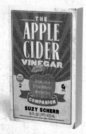 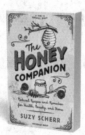 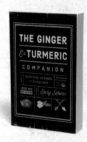

SUZY SCHERR is a chef, culinary instructor, and cookbook author whose work has appeared in *Rachael Ray Every Day*, on *The Today Show*, and elsewhere. She lives with her family in New York.

© Jamie Meadows

COOKING

Cover art: (olive leaves) L_G_Anna / Getty Images; (olives) aqua_marinka / iStock / Getty Images; (chips and sea salt) Daria Ustiugova / Shutterstock; (olive oil) Angry_red_cat / Shutterstock; (background) MM_photos / Shutterstock
Cover design: Allison Chi

THE COUNTRYMAN PRESS
A division of W. W. Norton & Company
www.countrymanpress.com

$14.95 USA $19.95 CAN.
ISBN 978-1-68268-630-0

5 1 4 9 5
9 781682 686300

Printed in the United States of America